Praise for *Dads Raising Children with Special Needs & Disabilities*

"This insightful and beautifully written book accurately captures the pain of mourning the life and potential we anticipated for our children with special needs and disabilities and highlights the fundamental importance of rediscovering life's simple but profound moments and truths through their eyes. While the power of family and community cannot be overstated, we must heed Hirsch's wisdom and look inward, allowing this experience to transform us into the strongest, kindest, most boundary-defying fathers we can be—staunch advocates, unwavering champions, and those who are not only willing to listen but capable of making others see and hear."

—Israel Defense Forces Maj. Gen. (Res.) Doron Almog, founder and chairman of the ADI Negev-Nahalat Eran Rehabilitation Village, 2016 Israel Prize Laureate, and chairman of the Executive of the Jewish Agency for Israel

"David Hirsch has written a book that feels like sitting with a wise friend who understands the real emotional terrain of raising a child with disabilities. As a father of an autistic adult child, I recognize the truth in these pages: the grief, the grit, and most importantly, the unexpected joy. David's blend of story, practicality, and wholehearted advocacy creates a roadmap rooted in dignity and love. A reassuring, steadying resource for any dad navigating a journey that reshapes you in all the important ways."

—Jonathan Bennett, executive coach, author, and proud father of two, Ontario, Canada

"Beyond brilliant. David's intellect and compassion combine to identify and illuminate fatherhood pathways that can sustain, even enrich, lives and loves of special dads and special kids. It's never easy, but striving is often its own reward."

—John Borling, retired US Air Force Major General, Vietnam Veteran, POW six years, eight months, author of *Taps on the Walls: Poems from the Hanoi Hilton*

"For any parent of a child with special needs, the journey ahead can feel incredibly daunting and even more so as a solo parent. Often, the role of the fathers in these situations can be overlooked or, perhaps more specifically, misunderstood. Through this book and via his charity, David provides invaluable support and guidance to fathers as well as sending a clear message that many are desperate to hear—that they do not have to face this alone."

—James Burch, Partner Walkers (Cayman) LLP, father of three

"David Hirsch delivers a powerful, practical, and deeply human guide for fathers on a journey few prepare for, but many are called to. As a father of a son with Down syndrome, I know how vital it is to hear from someone who's walked the path—and built community along the way. This book is equal parts compass and companion, offering wisdom, courage, and heart. A must read for every dad learning to redefine strength, hope, and what it means to lead with love."

—Mark X. Cronin, cofounder, John's Crazy Socks and Abilities Rising

"The No. 1 problem domestically facing America today is the breakdown of the family. A kid raised without a dad is five times more likely to be poor and commit crimes. Nine times more likely to drop out of school, and twenty times more likely to end up in jail. It is my firm belief David Hirsch has done more to bring the role of fatherhood to the forefront and its importance in our society than anyone in this country and maybe the world."

—Tom Dreesen, comedian, actor, and author

"This book strikes at the heart of what matters most—not just to families like mine, but to every family, community, and society that hopes to reach its potential and thrive."

—John F. Crowley, president and chief executive officer of Biotechnology Innovation Organization (BIO)

"This will become the foremost book for special needs dads, grounded in lived experience, deep research, and hundreds of honest father-to-father conversations."

—Reena Friedman Watts, Host of *Better Call Daddy* Podcast

"Good outcomes for children with special needs require practical thinking and involved parents. David Hirsch understands this, and his book gives fathers clear, usable guidance that truly helps families thrive."

—Temple Grandin, author of *Visual Thinking* and *Thinking in Pictures*

"This book is a must-read for all current and future fathers. It is an example of the joys and challenges of being a father. It shows why a father can learn as much from their kids as they can teach their children."

—Lon Haldeman, legendary pioneer of American ultradistance cycling

"David Hirsch is someone I have admired for years. Looking at abilities as opposed to disabilities is so much more impactful. This is a playbook and guide for every father to be his best. It will also provide you with the path to your own legacy."

—**Larry Kaufman, speaker, best-selling author of *The NCG Factor: A Formula for Building Life-Changing Relationships, from College to Retirement***

"David Hirsch has been an incredible mentor and friend, helping me establish the Special Fathers Network in Nairobi, Kenya. His guidance and leadership have inspired me and countless dads to embrace fatherhood with courage and love. As a father raising two children with special needs, I know firsthand the challenges and joys this journey brings. This book is a beacon of hope and practical wisdom—it will empower fathers everywhere to lead with resilience, compassion, and faith. David's work reminds us that we are never alone on this path."

—**Duncan Keya, Nairobi-based disability advocate and community organizer**

"Fatherhood is never a solo journey. This book reminded me how healing it is to share openly with other dads—the fears, the sleepless nights, the small victories that feel like miracles. In those conversations, I found strength, laughter, and the reassurance that none of us are alone. What matters most is knowing our children feel loved, safe, and accepted—and that we, as fathers, can lean on each other to make that possible."

—**Ágúst Kristmanns, Reykjavík-based disability advocate and father of three**

"A powerful collection of wisdom from fathers whose lives were forever changed by a child's diagnosis—offering practical guidance, honest compassion, and hope for the road through uncertainty, tears, and unexpected joy."

—**Randy Lewis, former executive vice president of Walgreens, author of *No Greatness Without Goodness***

*"I am excited to recommend **Dads Raising Children with Special Needs and Disabilities: A Guide for 21st Century Dads**. Many special needs dads feel lost, alone, and overwhelmed. Realizing that you are not alone is important. Each chapter has a special focus. Several focus on building dads on a personal level. Chapter 4's focus is 'Being Present: Physically, Emotionally, and Spiritually for Your Child,' while Chapter 6 focuses on 'Self-Care for Dads: Prioritizing Your Well-Being to Better Serve Your Family' and Chapter 11 focuses on 'Mastermind Groups: Tapping into Collective Wisdom and Support.' Each chapter will help dads become the best they can be."*

—**Allen Lynch, grandfather of child with special needs, Vietnam veteran, and Medal of Honor recipient**

"Being a father of a special needs child myself, it's gratifying to see that David Hirsch has once again taken the time and effort to provide yet another resource for us dads. I'm proud to have known David for decades and continue to applaud his commitment to this aspect of his life and those of us fathers."

—Joe Mantegna, award-winning actor on Broadway, television, movies, and the voice of Fat Tony on *The Simpsons*

"The subtitle of my best-selling book **Aspire!** *is* **How to Create Your Own Reality and Alter Your DNA***. David's new book* **Dads Raising Children with Special Needs and Disabilities** *goes beyond that. David's book actually changes the mind of fate itself by delivering a courageous, compassionate roadmap for fathers navigating life's toughest terrain. His wisdom encourages us to show up stronger, love deeper, and lead with intention. This book is a gift to dads everywhere and a triumph of purpose-driven living."*

—Frank McKinney, nine-time best-selling author in eight genres

"Life can change in a split second—mine did. David Hirsch understands what it means to keep showing up as a dad when everything feels different. His book gives fathers hope, direction, and strength when they need it most. It's heartfelt, practical, and written by someone who truly gets it."

—Jim Mullen, entrepreneur and disabled Chicago police officer (On October 17, 1996, Jim was catastrophically injured in the line of duty and became a ventilator-dependent quadriplegic. His daughter Maggie was 7 months at the time.)

"David Hirsch is the voice so many special needs fathers have been waiting for. In this book, he brings decades of lived experience, advocacy, and deep listening to the page with humility and clarity. David doesn't speak at fathers—he walks beside them. His wisdom is earned, his compassion is real, and his commitment to fatherhood is unwavering. This book captures the honesty, exhaustion, faith, humor, and fierce love that define the journey of raising a child with special abilities. If you're a dad navigating this path, David's words will reassure you that you're not alone—and that your presence truly matters."

—Brady Murray, father of ten, founder of RODS Heroes

"This book is a must read for all who are and aspire to be great fathers. It is an enlightening book about the challenges, ideas, solutions, joys, and celebrations of being a dad even in the most trying circumstances. It deals with specificity regarding the unique special needs of certain children and how we, as fathers, can help our children reach their full potential. Read this and you will be a better dad."

—Warren Rustand, husband, father, chief executive officer, speaker, and author, *The Leader Within Us*

"This insightful and heartfelt book is a gift to fathers of children with special needs. David brings wisdom, honesty, and deep compassion to every page, offering guidance that is both practical and uplifting. As a fellow advocate for families, I admire the strength and hope this work provides. His blend of personal experience, poetry, and even humor creates a meaningful companion for dads navigating their unique journey. I highly recommend it."

—Rabbi Kalman Samuels, cofounder of Shalva, the Israel Association for the Care and Inclusion of Persons with Disabilities, and author of *Dreams Never Dreamed*

"Life sparkles with blessings—a special blessing for me was the day I met David Hirsch.

"Where some see 'difference,' David sees that which is special. In a world that rigidly defines 'success,' David celebrates the individual. Where souls are burdened with the label of 'disability,' David's innate response is to love, to encourage, to support.

"This remarkable man, infused with seemingly boundless energy, wisdom, and drive, is a beacon of hope for so many—especially those of us who 'father children with special abilities!'

"It is a privilege to support his endeavors and to call him my friend."

—Dr. Shane Sondergeld, Brisbane, Australia

"I have known David Hirsch for a number of years and have been privileged to speak to his Special Fathers Network organization on multiple occasions. As a blind person myself, and as someone who grew up in a home with several special needs kids, I know the power of being influenced by a positive and encouraging dad. This book is a treasure for anyone who deals with or interacts with special needs kids. There's no greater way to make a huge difference where it is most needed, and David's book will equip you for the task."

—Jim Stovall, founder of Narrative Television Network, and best-selling author of *The Ultimate Gift*

"I believe that it is essential to honor those fathers who have taken on the challenge of providing unshakable love for their children who are facing difficult life challenges."

—Bill Strickland, founder of Bidwell Training Center and Manchester Craftsmen's Guild, author, and social entrepreneur

"This book is a heartfelt tribute to the courage, tenderness, and quiet heroism of fathers raising children with special needs. It captures how fatherhood transforms us—softening some parts, strengthening others—while teaching us to see possibility where the world sees limits. With practical guidance and deeply human insight, it shows how to build a fuller, more hopeful life, focusing on ability, dignity, and love. The chapter 'Cerebral Palsy and Strength' resonates with me profoundly as the father of a child with CP—it reflects our truth: Strength is not loud; it grows in everyday moments, in patience, and in unconditional devotion."

—Dr. Ruslan Vasyutin, Ukrainian dad, psychotherapist, coach, and social entrepreneur

Dads Raising Children with Special Needs & Disabilities

A Guide for 21st Century Dads

David Hirsch

Foreword by John F. Crowley

Copyright © 2026 David Hirsch

All rights reserved. No part of this book may be reproduced or transmitted in any form or by any means, electronic or mechanical, including photocopying, recording, or by any information storage and retrieval system, without permission in writing from the publisher.

Published by Transformation Media Books, USA

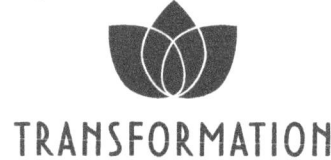

www.TransformationMediaBooks.com
info@TransformationMediaBooks.com
An imprint of Pen & Publish, LLC
Saint Louis, Missouri
(314) 827-6567
www.PenandPublish.com

Paperback ISBN: 978-1-956897-79-1
ebook ISBN: 978-1-956897-80-7
Library of Congress Control Number: 2026933633

Cover Design: Stacy Chambers, stacy@mergz.com
Mergz Media, LLC, https://mergz.com

Dedicated to my wife, Peggy; my children, Dave, Amanda, Emily, Charlie, and Addie, and future generations; as well as all the SFN Mentor Fathers and special needs parents, who are the real heroes in society.

Acknowledgments

This book represents more than a decade of listening to, learning from, and standing alongside fathers raising children with special needs and disabilities. While it carries one author's name, it reflects the collective wisdom, generosity, and courage of a global community. I offer my sincere gratitude to:

The **900+ SFN Mentor Fathers**, located across the United States and in more than a dozen countries worldwide: Thank you. You are the backbone of the Special Fathers Network. Your willingness to support other dads—often at the most vulnerable moments of their lives—through shared experience, empathy, and practical guidance is nothing short of extraordinary. You are too numerous to list individually, but your impact is profound and enduring.

My deepest appreciation to the **400+ *SFN Dad To Dad Podcast* guests**, listed in chronological order from episodes 1 through 420 in Appendix A. Each of you shared your heartfelt stories with honesty and courage, helping normalize conversations about fatherhood, disability, grief, resilience, marriage, advocacy, and hope. Your voices form a living oral history that directly informed this book.

Thank you to the **SFN Mastermind Group** dads (also listed in Appendix A) who make a weekly commitment of time and monthly investment to show up for one another. Your willingness to share wins, wrestle with challenges, reflect on books, and engage in deep, respectful conversation week after week exemplifies what healthy, intentional male community can look like. This book is stronger because of what I have learned from you.

I am grateful to the **21st Century Dads Foundation Board**, listed here for your leadership, stewardship, and guidance. Your belief in the mission, your strategic insight, and your willingness to lead have helped ensure that this work remains sustainable, credible, and impactful: **Tom Costello, Rich Gathro, Gary Grube, Christopher Hunter, Shane Madden, Wayne Messmer, Brian Page,** and **John Shouse.**

To the **individuals, families,** and **corporations** who have generously funded the 21st Century Dads Foundation and Special Fathers Network over the past decade: Thank you. Your early belief and continued support made it possible to build programming, produce content, convene communities, and reach fathers who otherwise might have remained isolated. This book is, in many ways, an extension of that shared investment.

Special acknowledgments for this book. Several individuals deserve recognition for their direct contributions to this project:

- **John Crowley**, friend, mentor, and arguably one of the most iconic rare-disease dads of all time, whose generosity and perspective are reflected in the Foreword. Your words set the tone for this book in a way only lived experience can.
- **Jennifer Geist**, of Transformation Media Books, our publisher, for her belief in this project and her steady guidance in bringing it to print.
- **Tom Couch**, my wingman with the *SFN Dad To Dad Podcast* for all but two of the first 420 episodes. Thank you for your partnership, your judgment, and for carefully selecting the audio clips used in the Audible edition and which appear in the print edition as quotes.
- **Janet Shouse**, of Franklin, Tennessee, for her extraordinary editorial work on the original manuscript. Your editing skills were remarkable, but your insight as the parent of an autistic adult son was invaluable. This book is clearer, stronger, and more grounded because of you.

Finally, this book is dedicated to all special needs dads and moms everywhere for being the real heroes of parenting. You are, on average, *more humble, less arrogant,* and *less selfish* than the overall population. Your role modeling is more important than you may ever know, so thank you.

—**David Hirsch**

Contents

Foreword by John F. Crowley	xiv
Preface	xix
1. Redefining Fatherhood: The Journey of Raising a Child with Special Abilities	1
2. Strength Through Unity: The Power of Marriage in Navigating Special Needs	7
3. Grieving the Life You Anticipated: Finding Peace in the New Reality	16
4. Being Present: Physically, Emotionally, and Spiritually for Your Child	27
5. Father-to-Father Mentoring: Wisdom, Support, and Strength in Community	40
6. Self-Care for Dads: Prioritizing Your Well-Being to Better Serve Your Family	51
7. Respite and Renewal: The Importance of Taking Breaks Without Guilt	63
8. Faith and Fatherhood: Spirituality as a Guide on the Special Needs Journey	73
9. Siblings Matter: Balancing Attention and Love Across the Entire Family	85
10. Family Leadership: Building a Strong, Healthy, and Unified Household with Vision, Intent, and Values	96
11. Mastermind Groups: Tapping into Collective Wisdom and Support	110
12. IEPs, Setting and Accomplishing Goals, and Celebrating Wins, Large and Small	121

13. Living in the Present: Thriving in the Circumstances You Didn't Expect	127
14. The Unwavering Commitment: 24/7/365 Fatherhood and What It Really Takes	138
15. Fostering Independence and Self-Sufficiency: Helping Your Child Build Confidence, Find Purpose, and Gain Employment	149
16. Protecting Your Family: The Importance of Estate and Financial Planning	159
17. Dads Raising Children with Autism: Navigating a Unique Path with Love and Patience	168
18. Supporting Children with Down Syndrome: Focusing on Abilities, Not Limitations	177
19. Rare Diseases and Resilience: Adapting to the Unknown with Courage	186
20. Cerebral Palsy and Strength: Overcoming Challenges with Determination	198
21. The Legacy of Fatherhood: Leaving a Lasting Impact on Your Family and Community	204
Epilogue: Embracing the Journey of Fatherhood	214
Curriculum: A Resource for Further Reflection	C1
Appendix A: Books and 21CD Resources	265
Appendix B: A Primer of Additional Resources for Parents Raising Children with Special Needs and Disabilities	273

Foreword

When you spend your professional life in biotechnology, you become accustomed to thinking about systems—biological systems, regulatory systems, innovation ecosystems. But fatherhood, especially fatherhood in the world of rare diseases and disabilities, teaches you to think about systems at a much more personal level. It teaches you to see the human beings within those systems—young children fighting for their lives, families navigating complex medical, educational, and emotional landscapes, and fathers deciding, every single day, whether they will step forward or step away.

For me, fatherhood has been the most consequential leadership role of my life. It has shaped my priorities, defined my values, and guided every major professional decision I've made—from joining the Navy, to building a biotech company to save my children's lives, to advocating in our nation's capital for policies that advance more cures and treatments for patients and families in need.

That is why I am honored to write this foreword for David Hirsch's extraordinary book, ***Dads Raising Children with Special Needs and Disabilities: A Guide for 21st Century Dads***. This book strikes at the heart of what matters most—not just to families like mine, but to every family, community, and society that hopes to reach its potential and thrive.

It speaks with clarity and compassion about the essential role fathers play, especially when life veers sharply from the expectations we once held. And it provides the kind of thoughtful, experience-based guidance that modern dads desperately need, but too rarely receive.

The Father Who Shaped Me

I learned much of what I know about fatherhood from my own dad, John Crowley. He was a man of quiet strength—disciplined, principled, and profoundly committed to his family. He served as a US Marine and carried the weight of that experience with dignity. He worked long hours and faced hardships that I only came to fully understand as an adult, yet he always made time for us. Very sadly, he lost his life when I was 7 years old, while serving as a New Jersey police officer. The trauma of growing up without my dad and watching my mom struggle to raise me and my brother would have a huge impact on me and my future.

Those lessons rooted deep, but I don't think I appreciated their full significance until the moment two of my children—our daughter, Megan, and our son Patrick—were diagnosed with Pompe disease. Suddenly, the abstract ideals of what it means to be a father became urgent, concrete responsibilities. The stakes were no longer conceptual. They were life or death.

In the years that followed, as my wife and I navigated the scientific, logistic, emotional, and spiritual challenges of raising children with a life-threatening rare disease, I understood something essential: Fatherhood is not a title. It is a mission.

And it is a mission that requires intentionality, fortitude, humility, and community.

Why a Father's Involvement Matters—More Than Ever

Research on child development is unequivocal: Children do better when their fathers are involved. When fathers step forward, their kids demonstrate stronger emotional health, better academic outcomes, and higher resilience.

But for children with disabilities or complex medical needs, a father's involvement becomes even more critical.

These families often face frequent medical appointments, navigating multiple specialists and educational advocacy challenges, as well as financial strain, emotional uncertainty, and social isolation.

When fathers are engaged—emotionally, mentally, spiritually—the family becomes stronger. Marriages are more resilient. Siblings feel more supported. A child with special needs has the advocates they need on multiple fronts.

Yet we still live in a culture where mothers are expected to be the primary caregivers, and fathers are often relegated to supporting roles. That model is outdated, unsupported by evidence, and harmful to families.

What David offers in this book is not merely encouragement for dads to "get more involved." He offers more—a framework for what involvement *looks like*—how to approach it with intention, how to sustain it over time, and how to grow into the father your child needs, even when the journey tests you in ways you never anticipated. In the world of science and policy, we often talk about "evidence-based practices." David's work is evidence-based fatherhood.

Intentionality: The Leadership Discipline That Begins at Home

I have spent much of my professional life leading organizations through uncertainty—biotech startups, global patient advocacy initiatives, and now the world's premier biotechnology trade association. Through it all, I've learned that leadership requires clarity of purpose, steadiness under pressure, and the ability to chart a course through rapidly changing circumstances.

But fatherhood—especially fatherhood in a family with special needs—requires all of that and more. It requires intentionality.

Intentionality means choosing not to be passive.

Intentionality means refusing to let circumstances dictate your role.

Intentionality means showing up fully, even when you feel depleted.

It means listening deeply to your child, learning the complexities of their condition, and advocating in medical settings, as well as supporting your partner, balancing high-stakes decisions with compassion, and being present when the emotional weight is heavy.

In my own life, intentionality meant leaving a stable corporate career to pursue life-saving treatments for my children, even when the odds of success were long. It meant building a biotechnology company anchored in purpose. It meant fighting through scientific setbacks, organizational challenges, and legal battles. It meant knowing that the stakes were too high to sit on the sidelines. Time was too precious to wait.

And it meant doing all of this while still being Dad—showing up for bedtime, for birthdays, for school events, for quiet moments of fear and hope. For a late kiss goodnight.

Intentional fatherhood is not about perfection. It's about prioritization. It's about aligning your actions with your deepest values.

This book gives fathers the tools to do exactly that.

Living a Life of Purpose: Our Children as Guides

I sometimes think that the clearest view of human potential comes not from boardrooms or laboratories, but from hospital rooms and therapy centers—from the quiet places where children fight for each small victory, where parents celebrate milestones that others take for granted, and where love becomes a force more powerful than fear.

My children have taught me more about purpose than any professional accomplishment ever could. Watching Megan and Patrick persevere through a debilitating condition like Pompe disease has taught me about the tremendous nature of human resilience. Along with my son John Jr., they have also taught me gratitude, to see ability where others see limitation, and to hope boldly.

These are lessons deeply embedded in the fabric of this book.

The fathers you will meet in these pages—through David's interviews, stories, and reflections—have walked roads that require courage, wisdom, humor, and faith. Their experiences form a kind of collective intelligence—an accumulated wisdom that can guide new fathers facing their own uncertainties.

David has curated and distilled that wisdom with remarkable clarity. His work honors the challenges families face, but it also celebrates the love and joy that define this journey.

This is not a book about hardship. It is a book about strength.

It is not a book about limitation. It is a book about potential.

It is not a book about diagnoses. It is a book about identity, meaning, and hope.

Why This Book Matters—Now More Than Ever

We are living in a time of unprecedented scientific progress. Gene therapies, personalized medicine, AI-driven discoveries—these innovations offer hope that would have been unimaginable a generation or two ago. As CEO of BIO, I see this progress every day.

But scientific breakthroughs are only part of the equation. Families need emotional, relational, and social breakthroughs as well. They need models of engaged fatherhood. They need tools to navigate complex systems. They need communities that sustain them.

David's work fills a gap that science cannot fill: the gap of human connection.

He reminds us that no medical advancement can replace the steady, loving presence of a father. No scientific achievement can substitute for the hope a child feels when their dad believes in them.

And no policy change—however important—can replace the ripple effects of a father's daily, intentional decisions to show up for his child.

This book strengthens the foundation upon which families build their futures. It elevates fathers as essential partners in caregiving, not secondary participants. It provides guidance that is practical without being prescriptive, honest without being discouraging, hopeful without being naive.

It is a manual for modern fatherhood.

A vision for what is possible.

And a testament to the extraordinary power that resides in everyday acts of love.

Closing Thoughts

When I look back on my own journey—the uncertainty, the challenges, and eventually, the breakthroughs—I see a pattern I could not fully appreciate in the moment. I see how every act of fatherhood, from the smallest gesture to the largest sacrifice, became part of a larger narrative of love and determination.

I see how my own father's example prepared me for a future neither of us could have imagined.

I see how the resilience of my children reshaped my understanding of leadership and strengthened my resolve.

And I see how the support of community, science, faith, and family made the impossible possible.

What David Hirsch has created in this book is a roadmap for fathers just beginning their own journeys—and a companion for those who have been on the road for years. It is filled with wisdom, empathy, and practical insight. It is grounded in research but elevated by lived experience. It calls fathers to rise with intention, lead with heart, and love with steadfastness.

For every father holding a diagnosis in one hand and doubt in the other, this book is a lifeline. For every dad who feels isolated, overwhelmed, or unsure, it is a reminder that he is not alone. And for every child whose life will be shaped by the devotion of a caring, committed father, it is a promise that their journey matters.

It is my honor to recommend this book to every father, every family, and every community that wants to build a future defined not by limitations, but by possibilities.

—John F. Crowley
Chief Executive Officer, Biotechnology Innovation Organization (BIO)
Former CEO & Executive Chairman, Amicus Therapeutics
Rare-disease advocate
Proud father of three

Preface

While I'm the father of five adult children ranging in age from 29 to 36 and have been an outspoken advocate for father involvement for nearly three decades, the experiences that shaped my understanding of fatherhood date back to when I was in first grade. My parents divorced when I was six and my younger brother, Ronald, was five. All I understood then was that my dad moved away, got remarried, and became a dad to someone else's kids.

As a young boy, I remember the police being involved when my dad would show up unannounced and refuse to leave, forcing my mom to call for help. I also remember having to go downtown to the Daley Center, the huge courthouse in Chicago, Illinois, to attend court appearances. We had to move in with my grandparents which necessitated changing schools. My mom, Claire, was our primary (and for the most part sole) caregiver and parent for the next seven years. She did the best she could as a Chicago Public Schools teacher who taught special education during the last decade of her three-decade career. I think part of her compassion for teaching special education stemmed from the fact my brother had an Individualized Education Program (IEP). I share some of these details, not for sympathy or pity, but to emphasize that there were not a lot of resources for our family, and especially because my dad was reluctant to adhere to the court order for child support and alimony. I didn't spend much time with my dad from the time I was 6 until I was 13.

Thank God for my maternal grandfather, Sam Solomon, who became my primary father figure when I was 6 and until he passed away at age 93 in 2001, when I was 40 years old. We shared a very special relationship. I was the first of his three grandchildren and was born on his birthday, so we always celebrated our birthdays together.

Through some extreme circumstances my brother and I ended up living with my dad and stepmom. Looking back, it was a challenging situation and only became more dysfunctional as time went by. There was about a ten-year period when I was 21 to 31 that I had almost zero contact with my dad. For more details you can go to Chapter One in my first book, *21ˢᵗ Century Dads: A Father's Journey to Break the Cycle of Father Absence*.

When I became a father, I had a clear idea of the type of dad I wanted to become. I was intent on emulating those who got it right, like my Grandpa Sam, and avoiding the mistakes I saw others, like my dad, make. If that sounds hard-hearted or disrespectful, it's simply the truth.

Dads Raising Children with Special Needs and Dis**abilities** is the product of two overarching experiences. First, I've been an outspoken advocate for father involvement since founding the Illinois Fatherhood Initiative (IFI) in 1997, whose mission is "actively engaging fathers in the educational lives of their children." The signature program of IFI is an essay-writing program that has involved more than 425,000 school-age children writing essays to the theme "What My Father Means to Me." That included an appearance on *The Oprah Winfrey Show*, the involvement of hundreds of Illinois schools, hundreds of volunteer evaluators each year, an *Essay Booklet* with a curriculum, and three fatherhood celebrations each year for more than two decades. The big takeaway? When fathers are actively engaged in the educational lives of their children, educational outcomes go up dramatically, and many of society's greatest challenges—including crime and incarceration, drug and alcohol abuse, and teen suicide and pregnancy—go down dramatically. Simply put, greater father involvement equals greater student achievement. In other words, your children benefit and so does society at large.

Second, through founding and leading the 21ˢᵗ Century Dads Foundation (21CD) the past ten years, I've seen the devotion and persistence of fathers who have children with disabilities or special health-care needs. The signature program of 21CD is the Special Fathers Network (SFN), a dad-to-dad mentoring program with more than nine hundred SFN Mentor Fathers, most of whom have more than ten years of experience raising children with disabilities. Along the way and quite unexpectedly, I became the host of the *SFN Dad To Dad Podcast*, now with more than four hundred weekly episodes. The goal of the podcast has been to shine a bright light on the positive aspects of raising children with special health-care needs and disabilities, while not shying away from the day-to-day realities and challenges.

21CD has also birthed a YouTube channel and has created a series of audiobooks, including topics on autism, Down syndrome, rare disease, cerebral palsy, and on losing a child, that can be found on Audible. 21CD also hosts a growing number of SFN Mastermind Groups, which are small groups of fathers who have children with disabilities that meet virtually on a weekly basis. These sacred weekly meetings provide dads with a safe, judgment-free space to share wins, read and reflect on six books a year, and have discussions about the day-to-day challenges related to disability, their kids, their marriages, and their health, all capped off with the annual in-person SFN Mastermind Group Dads Weekend Retreat.

Over the past eight years, I have been reminded daily of the complex yet beautiful journey that many fathers embark upon while raising children with special abilities. This book is not merely a collection of chapters; it is a heartfelt exploration of the profound experiences, challenges, and triumphs that fathers face while navigating the often-uncharted waters of fatherhood in this context. It is a labor of love, shaped by the voices of fathers who have walked similar paths and have emerged with stories of resilience, hope, and unwavering dedication.

As a nationally recognized fatherhood advocate and host of the *SFN Dad To Dad Podcast*, I have had the privilege of taking a deep dive with hundreds of fathers from diverse backgrounds, each with their unique stories and struggles. Their experiences have painted a vivid picture of fatherhood that goes beyond traditional notions. It has opened my eyes to the reality that raising a child with special health-care needs or disabilities is not solely about managing challenges; it is about celebrating abilities, fostering growth, and cherishing every moment that comes with this extraordinary journey.

This book is structured into twenty-one chapters, each designed to address various aspects of fatherhood as it pertains to children with special abilities. The chapters are informed by personal stories, practical advice, and a deep understanding of the emotional landscape fathers traverse. They explore the redefinition of fatherhood, highlighting the unique dynamics that come into play when raising a child who may not fit the mold of what society typically expects or the vision you might have had before becoming a father.

As is the custom with our SFN Mastermind Groups, we start and end each weekly meeting on a positive note. Each chapter includes a brief father's poem to set the right tone for the subjects being discussed. On a lighter note, and with apologies to my children and wife, each chapter ends with a dad joke.

Sprinkled throughout this book are the actual heartfelt words excerpted from some of the four hundred-plus episodes of the *SFN Dad To Dad Podcast*. If you're listening to the audio version of this book, you're in for a real treat as you'll hear their actual voices.

As you journey through this book, I encourage you to reflect on your own experiences, challenges, and triumphs. Remember that you are not alone, unless you choose to be. No need to try to figure it out on your own, to resist the urge to pull over and ask for directions. The stories shared within these pages are testaments to the strength of fatherhood and the incredible ability of parents to adapt, learn, and grow alongside their children.

This book is a call to action for fathers everywhere—to embrace their roles, seek support, and celebrate the incredible abilities of their children. May it serve as a guiding light on your journey, providing wisdom, comfort, and inspiration as you navigate the remarkable path of parenting children with special needs and abilities. Together, let us redefine fatherhood, uplift one another, and champion the extraordinary capabilities that lie within each of our children.

Fact—parents (moms and dads) raising children with disabilities and special health-care needs are more humble, less arrogant and less selfish than parents in general. God only knows, we all need more people with humility and fewer who are arrogant and selfish.

Welcome to this transformative journey. As I'm often quoted as saying, "Life is a journey, enjoy the ride." Let's make the most of our fatherhood journey.

- 1 -
Redefining Fatherhood: The Journey of Raising a Child with Special Abilities

STRENGTH IN SMALL STEPS

Each step you take, though small it seems,
Is a giant leap beyond my dreams.
Your hands in mine, we face the fight,
Through darkest days and brightest light.

They said you'd struggle, that much is true,
But they don't see the strength in you.
And as you grow, I've come to find,
Your heart is stronger than the mind.

Fatherhood is often imagined as a series of milestones—the first steps, the first words, teaching life's lessons, and preparing a child for the world. But what happens when the journey doesn't follow the expected path? When you become a father to a child with special needs or disabilities, that imagined future may shift. Yet with that shift comes a new perspective on fatherhood—one that isn't defined by limitations, but by possibilities, resilience, and unique joys. This is the essence of *redefining fatherhood*.

In this chapter, we'll explore what it means to embrace a new narrative of fatherhood. You are not simply raising a child with special needs; you are nurturing abilities that may not be obvious to the world but are powerful and unique. Your child's abilities, talents, and potential can be cultivated with love, patience, and understanding. By shifting focus from what society often labels as "deficits" to what your child *can* do, you lay the foundation for a deeper, more meaningful relationship.

The Unexpected Gift of Fatherhood

For many fathers, receiving a diagnosis like autism, Down syndrome, cerebral palsy, or a rare disease is overwhelming. You may grieve the life you had envisioned for your child and your family, feeling unsure of how to move forward. These feelings are valid, but what lies beyond them is the realization that fatherhood is a gift—one that offers the opportunity to love unconditionally, to learn patience, to truly understand the value in people's differences, and to become an advocate for someone who sees or experiences the world differently.

The journey often begins with grief as you find your life and your child's life is very different from what you probably imagined fatherhood would be like. Most fathers work through the various stages of grief, which don't come in a particular order, but generally end up—after months or years—at acceptance. The acceptance is not just of your child's diagnosis or diagnoses, but of your evolving role as a father. In this new role, you'll find yourself wearing many hats: caregiver, teacher, protector, advocate, and most importantly, a source of love and stability. Your child's needs may be different, but the essence of fatherhood remains the same—guiding, nurturing, and helping your child grow to their fullest potential.

Focusing on Abilities, Not Just Disabilities

It's easy to get caught up in the challenges that come with raising a child with special needs. The world may present you with a list of what your child *can't* do, but your role as a father is to discover and nurture what your child *can* do. Every child, regardless of their diagnosis, has strengths, talents, and abilities waiting to be unlocked. It could be a unique way of communicating, their extraordinary attention to detail, or a passion for a specific activity. Our job as fathers is to help our children recognize and cultivate these strengths.

This requires a shift in mindset—one that rejects societal limitations and instead embraces the potential that lies within your child. It's about recognizing the victories that others might overlook and celebrating the milestones that others often take for granted. As you embrace this perspective, you'll find that your child's journey is one of incredible growth, not just for them, but for you as well.

The Evolution of Fatherhood

Redefining fatherhood is also about redefining yourself. The journey of raising a child with special needs challenges you to grow, to be more present, more patient, and more resilient. It pushes you to examine your own expectations, to let go of the pressure to meet societal norms, and to embrace a fatherhood that is deeply personal and meaningful.

You'll find yourself learning from your child in ways you never expected. Perhaps you'll learn the value of slowing down, of appreciating the small moments. Maybe you'll discover new ways to communicate, to connect on a deeper level. Through the challenges, you'll gain a deeper understanding of what it means to be a father, not just to a child with special needs, but to any child. Fatherhood, at its core, is about love, connection, and growth—both for your child and for yourself.

The Road Ahead

As we embark on this journey together, this book will offer guidance, insights, and encouragement for navigating fatherhood in a way that focuses on abilities. From strengthening your marriage and nurturing family balance to finding support through mastermind groups and mentors, you'll gain tools and strategies to thrive in this role. Along the way, you'll also be reminded to celebrate the wins—big or small—because every step forward is a victory.

This first step, however, begins with redefining what it means to be a father. It's not about fitting into a preconceived mold; it's about creating your own path and leading your child with love, strength, and unwavering commitment. You may not have chosen this journey, but it is yours—and within it lies the power to transform your child's life and your own.

Fatherhood in the context of raising a child with special needs is not a detour. It's a reimagined path that leads to greater understanding, deeper love, and ultimately, a more fulfilling relationship with your child. Embrace the journey, and you will find that the rewards are far greater than you ever imagined.

Some extraordinary examples of overcoming adversity gleaned from more than four hundred *SFN Dad To Dad Podcast* interviews include:

John Borling, a retired major general in the US Air Force, who flew ninety-six successful combat missions in Vietnam before being shot down and taken prisoner, when his first daughter was 7 months old. He was released from the notorious prisoner of war camp known as the Hanoi

Hilton after being held as a POW for more than six years. John went on to serve for thirty-seven years in the US Air Force. John's story emphasizes the importance of resilience.

> *The Texans wanted to do something small for you, so they had this party in the Cotton Bowl. And I can remember talking to the governor of Texas. He said, "Look, this is going to be low-key. Son, this is about as low-key as we Texans get."*
>
> *And, you know, Nixon did the big party at the White House in May of '73, where they gave us the run of the place.*
>
> —**John Borling**, *Dad To Dad Podcast*, **episode #307**

James Burch, a British attorney with the international law firm Walkers in the Cayman Islands, whose firstborn, Archie, needed to be medevaced to Miami, Florida, the day after his birth. The day before, James and his wife, Gemma, were walking along Seven Mile Beach, contemplating the parenting journey ahead. Because of the severity of Archie's situation, a previously undetected heart defect combined with unexpected delays in the delivery, they found themselves in the neonatal intensive care unit at Miami Children's Hospital. After several operations, the doctors were able to stabilize Archie, only to learn there was literally no brain activity. This was just the beginning of their surreal experience. Because of how US health care is funded and after blowing through their savings, the couple was forced to move to London where Archie would be able to receive the life-saving treatments he needed. The couple would not return home to the Cayman Islands for three years. James's story is an extreme example of dealing with your world being turned upside down.

> The doctor said, "I've seen kids with full brain activity—absolutely fine—have a very poor standard of life in the future. Something horrible happens." He said, "I've also seen children like Archie live very full, happy lives."
>
> He said, "My suggestion to you, as somebody now who is telling you that Archie is going to be in your life forever—and you're his parents and you're going to love him—is don't bother with neurology anymore. Literally just face into each day as it comes. Whatever challenges come, you'll deal with them. But when it comes to matters of the brain, we're only guessing. We don't know."
>
> And that stuck with me forever. It was a doctor called Dr. Rossi. If he ever hears this—thank you, Dr. Rossi.
>
> But we said, "Okay," and we just stopped. And in those moments, you're feeling very sorry for yourself. I think now, if I could go back in time and see the James and Gemma who were standing in that room there, with Archie now, it would be amazing. I don't think I would believe it.
>
> To say, "Well, this is Archie now—he's supporting his football team, doing this, playing sport. He's huge. He's a big 14-year-old boy, being a typical teenager who will be really annoying you because of his teenage ways." You wouldn't believe it.
>
> —**James Burch**, *Dad To Dad Podcast*, **episode #366**

Kalman Samuels is a rabbi and father of seven in Jerusalem, Israel. The Samuels' family life changed overnight when their second child, son Yossi—until then a typical, healthy 1-year-old child—unknowingly received a tainted batch of vaccines. Within twenty-four hours, Yossi went blind and deaf, plunging the family into shock, grief, and a medical mystery no one would acknowledge. What followed was not only a fight for their son, but a nine-year battle against institutions that refused to admit wrongdoing or accept responsibility. As Yossi's world went dark and silent, his parents refused to let his life be defined by disability or invisibility. With virtually no services available for children with severe disabilities, they began creating what did not exist. That journey led to the creation of Shalva, a globally recognized beacon of hope, delivering world-class disability services on a five-acre campus in downtown Jerusalem, serving thousands of children, adults, and families each year through early intervention, education, therapy, residential care, employment training, and family support—impacting lives across Israel and inspiring inclusive models worldwide. The Samuels' story is a story about social justice.

> *This was put to me by my sister. When we first moved to New York, she was there for a conference, and she said something very simple to me. She said, "Sit down, kid brother. The problem is not with your son. The problem is with you.*
>
> *"You're still dreaming he's going to be a ballplayer. He's going to play sports. You're still dreaming he's going to be a rabbi. He's not going to play sports, and he's not going to be a rabbi. But you've got to change the yardstick."*
>
> *Meaning you have to measure his successes with his yardstick, not with yours—so that if he does whatever it might be, on a seemingly small scale, for him, that might be more than winning the gold medal in the 100 meters at the Olympics.*
>
> —Kalman Samuels, *Dad To Dad Podcast*, episode #210

Be sure to check out Kalman's book, *Dreams Never Dreamed: A Mother's Promise That Transformed Her Son's Breakthrough into a Beacon of Hope*.

Conclusion: The Special Needs Journey

In a rather profound way, a month does not go by without my hearing a dad say,

> *"I would not have asked for a child with special needs, but knowing everything I know today, I would not change a thing."*

It's my hope that you will also think and believe the same.

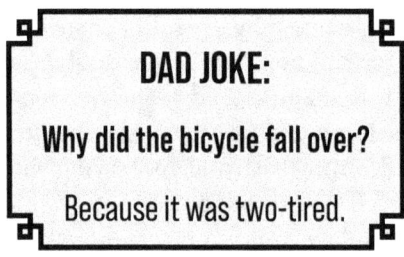

DAD JOKE:

Why did the bicycle fall over?

Because it was two-tired.

- 2 -
Strength Through Unity: The Power of Marriage in Navigating Special Needs

WE'RE IN THIS TOGETHER

Through sleepless nights and battles fought,
Through lessons time and trials brought,
I find my place, not just to guide,
But walk in faith, right by your side.

For marriage forged in love so true,
Is built on vows that we renew.
And fatherhood, a sacred call,
Is loving you—no bounds at all.

Disclaimer: My wife, Peggy, and I have been married for forty-two years in a heterosexual relationship. I also realize there are different family structures and a large number of special needs dads who either never married or are divorced. The term marriage and partnership are used here interchangeably to define the concept of coparenting. Also, for the single moms who might be reading or listening to this book, I have the utmost respect for the situation you find yourself in. I witnessed firsthand the struggles and sacrifices my mom made. She, like 99.99 percent of single moms, didn't plan to be a single mom. The decades of advocating for greater father involvement are in tribute to all the single moms, like my mom, who did (or who are doing) whatever it takes to help their children reach their full potential.

While not all children enter the world into two-parent families where the parents are married, I think it's important to recognize that marriage is a union built on love, trust, and shared goals. When a child with special needs or disabilities enters the picture, it can profoundly impact the marital relationship, challenging those foundations. However, rather than seeing these challenges as obstacles, couples who prioritize unity and communication can, with insight and grace, turn this experience into a source of deep strength and resilience.

The journey of raising a child with special needs is not just the child's journey; it's also the parents'. When parents come together, strengthening their marriage through shared understanding and support, they can create an unshakable foundation—not only for each other but also for the entire family. In this chapter, we'll explore the importance of maintaining a strong marriage while navigating the complexities of special needs parenting, and offer strategies for fostering connection, resilience, and unity in the face of life's challenges.

The Unique Strain of Special Needs on Marriage

Every marriage comes with its own set of challenges, whether it's managing finances, maintaining intimacy, or balancing work and family life, to name a few. But when a child with special needs is involved, those challenges can become magnified. Daily routines may often revolve around medical appointments, therapy sessions, and specialized care. This can lead to feelings of exhaustion, isolation, and overwhelm for partners.

It's no secret that the divorce rate among parents of children with special needs is higher than average. The added emotional, financial, and physical demands can strain even the strongest relationships. But it's important to remember that, despite the challenges, your marriage doesn't have to be a casualty of your circumstances. In fact, your relationship can become stronger and more resilient if you make the conscious choice to work together as a team.

Marriage as a Foundation for Resilience

A strong marriage can serve as the bedrock of stability and support in a family dealing with special needs. When couples are aligned in their purpose and commitment, they create a sense of security not only for themselves but also for their child and other family members. A united front can tackle problems more effectively and provide a buffer against the external pressures that inevitably arise.

But how does one foster such resilience in a marriage? It begins with a shared understanding that you and your spouse are in this together. You are each other's greatest ally in navigating the world of special needs, and maintaining a strong partnership will provide the stability your family needs to thrive.

Communication: The Lifeblood of a Strong Marriage

The foundation of any strong marriage is communication, but this becomes even more critical when parenting a child with special needs. Open, honest dialogue helps couples share their frustrations, fears, and hopes, and allows them to solve problems together.

1. **Create a Safe Space for Emotional Honesty:** In a relationship under stress, partners can sometimes retreat into their own emotional worlds, feeling isolated or misunderstood. It's vital to create a safe, judgment-free space where both partners can express their feelings. Whether it's discussing the exhaustion of managing a therapy schedule, the grief of unmet expectations, or the joy of witnessing a small victory in your child's development, emotional transparency is key.
2. **Listen with Empathy:** Effective communication is as much about listening as it is about speaking. When your spouse shares their feelings, listen with empathy. Instead of jumping to solutions or dismissing their concerns, acknowledge their emotions. Sometimes, simply being heard and understood can alleviate a great deal of stress.
3. **Make Time for Regular Check-Ins:** Life can feel like a whirlwind when raising a child with special needs, but setting aside time for regular check-ins is crucial. Whether it's a ten-minute conversation before bed or a weekly "marriage meeting," these check-ins provide an opportunity to assess how you're both feeling, express concerns, and ensure you're on the same page.

Shared Responsibilities and Teamwork

Parenting a child with special needs often requires juggling an overwhelming number of responsibilities. Medical appointments, therapies, school meetings, and day-to-day caregiving can quickly consume all your time and energy. One of the most important ways to foster unity in marriage is by sharing these responsibilities equitably.

1. **Divide Tasks Based on Strengths:** One effective strategy is to divide responsibilities based on each partner's strengths. If one of you is better at managing logistics like scheduling and paperwork, while the other excels at hands-on caregiving or attending medical appointments, play to those strengths. This not only helps manage

the workload but also makes both partners feel equally involved and valued.
2. **Avoid the Trap of Scorekeeping:** In times of stress, it's easy to fall into the trap of keeping score—mentally tallying who did what and feeling resentment when the balance seems off. But scorekeeping can quickly erode unity in a marriage. Instead, approach tasks as part of a shared goal: the well-being of your child and family. A mindset of collaboration over competition can make all the difference.
3. **Ask for Help and Accept It:** It's essential to recognize that you and your spouse don't have to do it all alone. Whether it's reaching out to extended family, hiring a respite care provider, or joining support groups, accepting help can relieve pressure on both partners. Asking for help is not a sign of weakness; it's a way to ensure your marriage and family remain healthy and balanced. Remember, speaking for all men, we're the gender that doesn't pull over and ask for directions. Don't be "that guy."

The Importance of Intimacy and Connection

Amid the demands of caring for a child with special needs, it's easy to lose sight of your relationship as a couple. Intimacy, both emotional and physical, often takes a back seat to the pressing needs of daily life. However, maintaining intimacy is essential to keeping your marriage strong and connected.

1. **Prioritize Quality Time Together:** Carve out time for just the two of you, even if it's just a few moments a day. Whether it's having coffee together in the morning, going for a walk, or scheduling a regular date night, these moments of connection remind you that you're not just coparents—you're also life partners.
2. **Reignite Physical Intimacy:** Physical intimacy can sometimes be one of the first casualties of a high-stress environment. But physical closeness, whether through simple touches, hugs, or sexual intimacy, plays a crucial role in maintaining connection. It's important to make time for these moments, even if it requires a bit of planning.
3. **Stay Emotionally Connected:** Beyond physical intimacy, emotional intimacy is what sustains a marriage during tough times. Try to stay emotionally connected by sharing your thoughts, dreams,

and fears with each other. The act of simply being there for one another, especially in times of difficulty, strengthens the emotional bond that will carry you through challenges.

Navigating Grief and Acceptance Together

One of the most profound challenges couples face when raising a child with special needs is coming to terms with grief—the grief of lost expectations, the grief of a future imagined but not realized. It's important to recognize that both partners may grieve differently. One spouse may feel sadness or anger, while the other might focus on acceptance or even optimism. These differences can create tension, but they can also be an opportunity for growth and understanding. Recognizing these differences and giving your partner some grace in this area goes a long way toward matrimonial harmony.

1. **Acknowledge Each Other's Grief:** Understand that your spouse may grieve in a way that's different from you, and that's okay. What's important is to acknowledge and respect each other's process. Grieving together can be a way of deepening your emotional connection and finding strength in each other.
2. **Move Toward Acceptance:** Over time, as you both process your grief, the goal is to move toward acceptance. Acceptance doesn't mean giving up or losing hope—it means finding peace with the reality of your child's needs while continuing to focus on their abilities and potential.
3. **Celebrate Your Child's Strengths:** A powerful antidote to grief is celebration. By focusing on your child's unique strengths and celebrating their achievements—no matter how small—you shift the focus from loss to possibility. Sharing in these moments of joy as a couple reinforces the positive aspects of your journey together.

Faith and Spirituality as a Source of Strength

For many couples, faith and spirituality play a significant role in their marriage and family life. When navigating the complexities of raising a child with special needs, faith can serve as a source of strength, comfort, and unity.

1. **Lean on Shared Spiritual Beliefs:** If you and your spouse share spiritual beliefs, leaning on those beliefs can provide a sense of

purpose and guidance. Prayer, meditation, or simply reflecting on your faith can help you find peace and resilience in times of uncertainty.
2. **Use Faith to Foster Gratitude:** Many spiritual traditions emphasize gratitude, which can be a powerful tool in reframing your experience as parents of a child with special needs. Focusing on the blessings in your life—your child's unique gifts, your spouse's support, the love that binds your family—can bring you closer together.
3. **Find a Faith-Based Support System:** Many faith communities offer support for families of children with special needs. Joining a group or finding spiritual mentors can provide a network of people who understand your challenges and can offer encouragement from a faith-based perspective.
4. **Are You the Faith Leader in Your Family?** I wasn't raised in a religious household. She is Catholic and I was Jewish. Since we were to be married in a Catholic church, we were required to go through pre-Cana, a form of premarital counseling. One condition was that if we have children, we were required to raise them as Catholics. For good or bad, it seemed like a small decision at the time. With the benefit of hindsight, I am very grateful for the leadership role my wife played in our family's religious life for the next twenty years.

Reflecting on the *SFN Dad To Dad Podcast* interviews, here are few dads with exemplary messages regarding the importance of marriage:

Brian Page of Orland Park, Illinois, who is the father of three, has a story that illustrates why marriage matters most when life turns unexpectedly hard. Their son Benjamin suffered a devastating brain bleed at birth that thrust the family into years of uncertainty, medical decisions, and emotional strain. Their marriage became the steady anchor that allowed their family not just to survive, but to grow stronger. Shared commitment meant shared burdens, mutual support, and the resilience to keep moving forward together. That same belief in strong families underpins Brian's work at Shepherds College, a three-year accredited residential program, where students thrive best when rooted in stable, loving homes. Marriage, in this light, is not optional—it is foundational.

> *And I said, "So, Dad, in some ways, Benjamin's kind of a miracle." And he said, "Well, you know, as physicians, we don't really use that terminology—but he's doing what he's not supposed to be doing."*
>
> *I think part of our perspective is that we're going to love him unconditionally and not put a ceiling over his life, and just have expectations that he was going to continue to grow and do everything that God really had for his life.*
>
> *He's now a student at Shepherds College. It was just overwhelming, in a positive sense, to walk around this campus—to see these other students who had a variety of special needs—and to know that there is something that someone thought of: a place like this, that our kid, whether he went there or not, could potentially do.*
>
> *I thought back to what the doctor had said: "Mr. Page, he's never going to walk." This kid is running a race—and he won the race.*
>
> —**Brian Page**, *Dad To Dad Podcast*, **episode #19**

Rick Bovell of Chicago, Illinois, is the father of five boys, including sons Evan and Daniel who are both autistic. Rick's life offers a powerful example of why marriage matters, especially in families touched by disability. Rick and his wife, Michelle, face daily demands that test patience, endurance, and faith. Marriage provides the stability that allows them to meet those challenges together—sharing responsibilities, supporting one another emotionally, and presenting a united front for their children. Their partnership makes space for grace when plans change and strength when fatigue sets in. Rick's active involvement with Joni and Friends, a global Christian disability ministry, reflects this same belief: strong marriages strengthen families. In the face of autism and uncertainty, marriage becomes not just a bond of love, but a lifeline.

> *Just a reminder for fathers: you are needed. Even if your wife is doing the lion's share of the work, be there for her. Don't feel as if she's got this. She doesn't have it without you.*
>
> —**Rick Bovell**, *Dad To Dad Podcast*, **episode #50**

Shane Sondergeld, a physician in Brisbane, Australia, who is the father of three, including a son with a rare genetic disorder, has found navigating complex medical care, advocacy, and the emotional weight of the unknown demands more than individual strength—it requires partnership. His son William has 4q deletion syndrome, and Shane has found marriage provides shared resolve, steady leadership, and the emotional ballast needed when one parent is exhausted or overwhelmed. In Shane's experience, a strong marriage creates stability for siblings, consistency for a child with complex needs, and hope for the future. Marriage becomes the structure that allows love, responsibility, and resilience to endure.

> *I look back on the times when I would always come in when he was ready to go to bed. I'd be there with him, and I'd talk to him. I'd tell him how much I love him. I'd read to him.*
>
> *I would make sure that we would always sit around the table at dinnertime to talk about the day—not sit in front of the TV. And I just think there are values you can bring to the relationship, but the most important one is love. Without all of this, it's clanging gongs. Love is the key to it all.*
>
> —**Dr. Shane Sondergeld**, *Dad To Dad Podcast*, **episode #72**

On the flip side, not all dads are married. While some were never married, others are divorced, and very sadly, some become solo dads as the result of their spouse passing away. That was the case with **Joe Ciriano**, whose life illustrates both the strength marriage provides and the void it leaves when lost. As a father of four in Burlington, North Carolina, Joe and his wife, Joy, built a marriage rooted in love, teamwork, and shared purpose while raising their children, including their daughter Grace, who has Down syndrome. For twenty-one years, their partnership sustained their family through daily challenges and quiet joys. When Joy tragically lost her battle with breast cancer, Joe was thrust into solo parenthood—carrying forward the values, resilience, and devotion they had built together. His journey shows that marriage is not only a source of strength in life, but a legacy that endures even in loss, guiding a family forward through love and faith.

> *Me, as a single father, having to deal with puberty with a developmentally disabled child. And both my older girls were gone. That was a challenge. That was a huge challenge and a fear from my perspective.*
>
> —Joe Ciriano, *Dad To Dad Podcast*, **episode #23**

Conclusion: The Power of a United Front

As you navigate the world of special needs parenting, remember that you are stronger together. A united partnership can serve as the foundation from which your entire family draws strength, stability, and love. By focusing on open communication, shared responsibilities, intimacy, and faith, you and your spouse can build a resilient partnership that supports your child's growth and nurtures your own.

In the end, a successful partnership is about navigating life's challenges together. And while the journey of raising a child with special needs may not have been the one you envisioned, it is one that can bring you closer as a couple. Together, you have the power to overcome obstacles, celebrate victories, and build a future filled with love and possibility for your family.

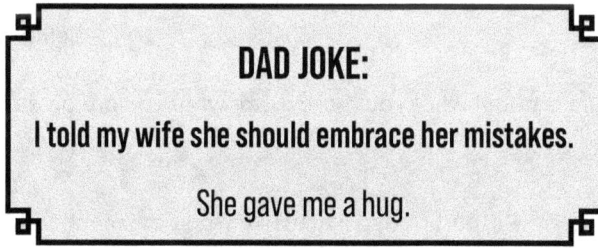

DAD JOKE:

I told my wife she should embrace her mistakes.

She gave me a hug.

- 3 -
Grieving the Life You Anticipated: Finding Peace in the New Reality

THE UNEXPECTED GIFT

I thought I knew what life would bring,
A child who'd run, a child who'd sing.
But life had plans beyond my own,
And gifted me a love unknown.

A love that teaches, shifts my view,
Reveals what's false, embraces true.
And though the road is steep and long,
With you beside me, I am strong.

"Life is not about what you have lost, but what you can still achieve."
—Jim Stovall

"The only thing you can control is your attitude.
It's all about your perspective."
—Bethany Hamilton

"Life is about what you make it, not what you are given."
—Coach Robert Mendez Jr.

The journey of fatherhood, particularly when raising a child with special needs, can be filled with immense joy and deep sorrow. While there are countless moments of love and connection, there often exists a quiet, painful undercurrent of grief for the life that was envisioned but may never come to fruition. This chapter delves into the grieving process, exploring how fathers can acknowledge and navigate their feelings of loss while finding peace in their new reality.

The Nature of Grief

Grief is a complex and multifaceted emotion. It is not simply a reaction to the loss of a loved one but can be a response to the many changes and challenges that accompany parenthood. In the context of raising a child with special needs, grief can arise from various sources.

Grieving Expectations. When a child is born, parents often hold dreams and expectations for their future, which may include aspirations for their child's education, friendships, milestones, and independence. When these expectations are challenged or altered, feelings of grief can emerge. **Example:** A father might have envisioned his child playing sports or attending a neighborhood school, only to find that his child needs additional support and accommodations, perhaps at a specialized school, to thrive. This shift can lead to feelings of loss for the anticipated experiences.

Grieving Identity. The identity of a father often evolves with the arrival of a child. When parenting a child with special needs, fathers may experience a shift in their sense of self and their role within the family. **Identity Changes:** Fathers may find themselves grappling with feelings of inadequacy, frustration, or confusion as they adapt to their new responsibilities and navigate the complexities of advocacy and care.

Grieving Relationships. The dynamics of relationships within the family can also shift when a child has special needs. Siblings may feel neglected, and the partnership between spouses may be strained as they navigate the challenges together. **Impact on Relationships:** Fathers might feel as though they are losing a connection with their partner or other children due to the demands of caregiving, leading to further grief and frustration. The stress of raising a child with special needs can take a toll on parental relationships, potentially leading to conflict or disconnection.

Acknowledging Grief

To find peace in the new reality, it is essential to acknowledge the feelings of grief rather than suppress them. This process can help fathers navigate their emotions in a healthy and constructive manner.

Allowing Space for Emotions. Grief is a natural response, and allowing oneself to feel these emotions is crucial. It is important to create a safe space where feelings can be expressed and explored without judgment.

One way to put grief into perspective is by journaling. Keeping a journal can serve as a therapeutic outlet for fathers to articulate their thoughts and feelings. Writing about grief can provide clarity and allow for reflection on the complexities of the journey. The Special Fathers Network has dozens of dads who started out journaling for their own peace of mind that led to sharing their insights with others through blogs, websites, and books. Some examples include:

- **Rob Gorski** of Canton, Ohio, who is the father of three boys on the spectrum and who have a wide range of other diagnoses. Rob's journaling led to *The Autism Dad* blog and website.

> *There are challenges. There are hardships. There is an infinite amount of sacrifice you're going to have to make. But the rewards are so profound.*
>
> *We try to live our lives the best we can within the circumstances we're in, and we teach our kids to do the same.*
>
> —Rob Gorski, *Dad To Dad Podcast*, episode #16

- **Matt Mooney** of Fayetteville, Arkansas, whose son Eliot was born with Trisomy 18 (or Edwards syndrome). Because of Eliot's fragile situation they celebrated each day as if it was his birthday, releasing a helium balloon outside. Very sadly, Eliot only lived ninety-nine days. Matt and his wife, Ginny, redirected their grief into 99 Balloons, a nonprofit dedicated to building inclusive communities so that every person with disability and their family can live a full life within relationships.

> *She walks all the time now. She communicates with a device. And even if she didn't, we would still love her.*
>
> *We're constantly trying to live out the lessons that Eliot's life taught us. She is an absolute joy. And we did not rescue Lena—she has most certainly rescued us.*
>
> —Matt Mooney, *Dad To Dad Podcast*, episode #37

- **Mark Maguire** of Atlanta, Georgia, whose son has Cri du Chat syndrome. Mark started journaling and blogging, which led to writing a number of books, including *Confessions of a Special Needs Dad*.

> *Some people say, "One day at a time." Some days, it's one hour at a time. Some days, it's 15 minutes at a time.*
>
> *That was some of the best advice I ever received when I was overwhelmed with sadness, grief, and anger. I had to pull it together and say,* **Okay—just make it through the next 15 minutes. You can do this.**
>
> —Mark Maguire, *Dad To Dad Podcast*, **episode #39**

- **Bo Bigelow** of Portland, Maine, whose daughter, Tess, has a rare genetic syndrome called USP7 and autism. As part of his therapy, Bo created the *Better Every Day Podcast*, where he has chronicled Tess's and the Bigelow family's journey for the past nine years. Bo, in collaboration with Daniel DeFabio, also created the Disorder Film Festival and Disorder Channel to provide venues for disability films and documentaries.

> *I created a blog post about Tess and included USP7—her symptoms, all of it. I took a deep breath and put it out there.*
>
> *Less than twenty-four hours later, I got an email from a man who said, "I work on the USP7 gene." He told us there were seven other known patients. And if Tess turned out to belong to this group, she would be the eighth known patient in the world.*
>
> —Bo Bigelow, *Dad To Dad Podcast*, **episode #51**

- **Josh Avis** of Redlands, California, who with his wife, Heather, have three adopted children, including two with Down syndrome. The couple channeled their energies into an Instagram account and podcast by the title *The Lucky Few* and Heather has written a book entitled *The Lucky Few: Finding God's Best in the Most Unlikely Places*.

> *We think life is going to be a certain way. Culture tells us it's a negative thing.*
>
> *But when you actually experience it—those of us who have children with Down syndrome—we realize it's not negative at all. We're actually the lucky ones. We're fortunate to live life differently, to see the beauty in it, and to truly see the humanity of our children.*
>
> —Josh Avis, *Dad To Dad Podcast*, episode #82

Seeking Support. Opening up to trusted friends and family members, seeking therapy, or joining a support group can help fathers process their grief. Sharing experiences with others who understand can create a sense of solidarity and connection. As highlighted in Chapter 11, consider joining an SFN Mastermind Group, a local group, or online support group for fathers raising children with special needs. Connecting with like-minded dads who share similar experiences can provide validation and encouragement.

The Journey of Acceptance

Acceptance is a crucial part of the grieving process. It involves coming to terms with the new reality and embracing the present moment without dwelling on what has been lost. While it's human nature to reflect on the past or contemplate what could have been, it's not healthy to dwell on "*could have*," "*should have*" or "*would have*" thinking. We can't change the past, so it's important to be in the present and try to influence the future.

Embracing the New Reality. Acceptance does not mean resigning oneself to the circumstances but rather acknowledging and embracing the current situation. This can lead to personal growth and a deeper connection with your child. Practicing mindfulness techniques can help fathers stay grounded in the present. Mindfulness encourages focusing on the current moment rather than getting lost in thoughts of the past or worries about the future.

Finding Joy in the Journey. Fathers can learn to find joy in the everyday moments of their child's life. By focusing on the unique strengths and abilities of your child, you can cultivate appreciation for the present.

Celebrating Milestones. Each milestone achieved, no matter how small, should be celebrated. Acknowledging progress reinforces a positive mindset and highlights the child's growth and development.

Lessons from Inspirational Figures. Many individuals have faced significant challenges in their lives and emerged with powerful messages about resilience and acceptance. Their stories serve as a testament to the strength of the human spirit and the potential for growth amid adversity.

- **Jim Stovall** of Tulsa, Oklahoma, started losing his sight as a teenager and went completely blind by age 29. Jim's first of more than sixty books is *You Don't Have to Be Blind to See*. Eight of his books have been made into major motion pictures. My favorite is *The Ultimate Gift*. Jim is also the founder of the Narrative Television Network, that allows many of the thirteen million blind and sight-impaired individuals in the US to enjoy movies. Despite the profound challenge of going blind, Jim became a successful entrepreneur, sought-after public speaker, and author, emphasizing the importance of attitude and perspective. Jim's journey teaches fathers that while they may grieve the life they anticipated, they still possess the power to create a fulfilling and meaningful life. By focusing on what can be achieved, dads can transform their children's experiences into opportunities for growth.

> *One of the most powerful influences in my life was a four-year-old boy who came into my life. For three years, he taught me the unadulterated wisdom of the ages.*
>
> *When it comes to that big dream—that calling in your life—the answer is always yes, you can. The dream would not have been placed there if you and I didn't have the capacity to achieve it.*
>
> *So the question is never* **can we?**
>
> *The question is* **will we?**
>
> *That is Christopher's enduring legacy to me.*
>
> —Jim Stovall, *Dad To Dad Podcast,* **episode #163**

- **Bethany Hamilton** of Lihue, Hawaii, is a professional surfer, who lost her arm in a shark attack in 2003 at age 13, but refused to let this tragedy define her. With the help of her father, **Tom**, Bethany returned to the sport she loved and became an inspiration to many. She went on to write ten books and is founder of the Beautifully Flawed Foundation, a nonprofit that produces events that inspire, shares stories of hope, and provides emotional support to traumatic amputees. Hamilton's story exemplifies the idea that the only thing we can control is our attitude. Fathers and children can take inspiration from her resilience and choose to approach their circumstances with positivity and determination.

One of my friend Noah's best friends was also a shark-attack survivor—his name is Mike Kutz. He lost his leg below the knee.

He was the first person Bethany talked to in the hospital, outside of our immediate family. And he gave her hope. He said, "I'm surfing again. I lost my limb—but you can do this."

That gave her a glimmer of hope.

—**Tom Hamilton**, *Dad To Dad Podcast*, **episode #158**

- **Coach Robert Mendez Jr.** of Saratoga, California, was born in 1989 without arms or legs. With the help of his father, **Robert Mendez Sr.**, and his family, Robert developed a love of sports and playing Madden Football. He parlayed his knowledge of football and passion for motivating others into a career coaching high school football, where he has inspired countless individuals through his dedication to coaching and mentoring. His story emphasizes that our circumstances do not define our potential. Mendez's commitment to helping young athletes succeed illustrates that, despite physical limitations, it is possible to make a significant impact on the lives of others. Fathers can find encouragement in his story and strive to create a legacy of love, strength, and support for their children.

> *Obviously it was a little shocking and there were jokes going around. Typical teenagers, you know, a guy with no arms or legs. Not a lot of people have seen that. If you're taken aback, that's just natural and that's human. But after the first two seconds, he's just a normal guy.*
>
> *I don't care how good you are. I don't care how experienced you are. You guys are going to do everything as a team.*
>
> *He may not look like a coach. He definitely acts like one.*
>
> *One thing I care about more than anything is being a family. That is one thing I take pride on. I love people. I love you. I love you. I love you. I love you.*
>
> —Robert Mendez Jr., *Dad To Dad Podcast*, **episode #58**

Building a New Vision for the Future

Once fathers acknowledge their grief and begin the journey of acceptance, they can start to build a new vision for their family's future. This vision should be grounded in love, resilience, and hope.

Setting New Goals. Creating new goals that align with the family's current reality can provide a sense of direction and purpose. These goals should be realistic and focused on the unique strengths and abilities of the child. Collaboratively setting family goals that include the child's interests and aspirations can foster a sense of belonging and inclusivity. These goals should celebrate the individuality of each family member.

Fostering Growth and Development. Investing in opportunities for growth and development can create a positive environment for both fathers and children. This may include pursuing therapies, hobbies, or educational opportunities that align with the child's strengths. Focus on teaching life skills that promote independence and self-sufficiency. Encouraging children to learn and grow fosters a sense of accomplishment and enhances their confidence.

Finding Peace amid Grief

Ultimately, finding peace amid grief involves embracing the journey of fatherhood, recognizing the challenges, and celebrating the joys. It is a continuous process that requires patience, self-compassion, and resilience.

Cultivating Mindfulness. Practicing mindfulness can help fathers navigate their emotions and find peace in the present moment. Mindfulness encourages self-awareness and acceptance, enabling fathers to be fully present with their children.

Mindful Parenting: Incorporate mindfulness techniques into parenting by being fully engaged during interactions with your child. This practice strengthens the father-child bond and enhances the overall parenting experience. Here are ten habits and practices to develop mindfulness for dads:

1. **Start the Day with Gratitude:** Begin each morning by reflecting on three things you're grateful for as a father. This sets a positive tone and cultivates appreciation for your role.
2. **Practice Deep Breathing:** Incorporate deep breathing exercises (e.g., inhale for four counts, hold for four, exhale for four) during moments of stress or when you're feeling overwhelmed. It helps ground you in the present.
3. **Mindful Listening:** When your children or partner speak, give them your full attention. Put away distractions and focus on their words, emotions, and body language.
4. **Schedule Daily Check-Ins:** Spend five to ten minutes reflecting on your day: How were you present with your children? What could you improve tomorrow? Journaling can enhance this process.
5. **Engage in Play:** Dedicate uninterrupted time to play with your kids. Allow their creativity and energy to guide the activity and embrace the moment without thinking about your to-do list.
6. **Model Mindfulness:** Practice what you want your children to emulate. Demonstrate patience, emotional regulation, and being fully present in your actions.
7. **Pause Before Responding:** When faced with challenges or emotional situations, pause for a moment to process your emotions before reacting. This reduces reactive behavior and enhances thoughtful responses.
8. **Meditate Regularly:** Even five to ten minutes of daily meditation can help calm your mind and foster awareness. Apps like Headspace or Calm can guide beginners.
9. **Take Nature Walks:** Go on nature walks with your family or alone. Pay attention to the sights, sounds, and sensations around you, and encourage your kids to do the same.

10. **Limit Technology:** Set boundaries around screen time for both yourself and your family. Create designated "tech-free" zones or hours to enhance family connection and presence.

These habits can help fathers build a deeper connection with their families, manage stress more effectively, and enjoy the journey of fatherhood with intention.

Embracing Community Support. Lean on the support of friends, family, and community. Sharing the journey with others can lighten the emotional load and create a sense of belonging. Consider reaching out to other fathers for support. Peer relationships can provide a valuable source of encouragement and understanding during difficult times.

Building and Creating Resilience

1. **Prioritize Self-Care:** Maintain physical health through regular exercise, balanced nutrition, and adequate sleep. Take time for hobbies or activities that bring joy and relaxation. (Read more about self-care in Chapter 6.)
2. **Practice Mindfulness:** Use mindfulness techniques such as meditation, deep breathing, or journaling to stay present and manage stress.
3. **Foster a Strong Support Network:** Build relationships with other dads, especially those in similar situations, for shared advice and camaraderie. Join support groups, like the Special Fathers Network, to connect with others who understand your journey.
4. **Set Realistic Goals:** Break larger challenges into manageable steps. Celebrate small victories to maintain motivation and optimism.
5. **Cultivate Optimism:** Focus on what can be controlled and let go of what cannot. Develop a habit of gratitude by identifying positives in daily life.
6. **Learn and Adapt:** Embrace challenges as opportunities for growth and learning. Reflect on past experiences to understand how you've successfully navigated difficulties before.
7. **Model Emotional Regulation:** Show children how to handle emotions constructively by doing so yourself. Practice patience and understanding, especially in tough situations.

8. **Stay Purpose-Driven:** Keep your role as a father at the forefront and let your love for your family guide your decisions. Reflect on the positive impact you have on your children's lives.
9. **Engage in Community Service:** Helping others fosters a sense of purpose and builds empathy. Involve your children in activities that teach resilience through giving back.
10. **Seek Professional Support When Needed:** Don't hesitate to seek help from counselors, therapists, or life coaches if facing significant challenges. Be proactive in addressing mental health and stress management.

Developing resilience is a journey. It takes intentional effort but empowers dads to better handle the ups and downs of parenting, especially when raising children with unique needs.

Conclusion: A Journey of Resilience

Grieving the life anticipated is, for many, a key part of the journey of fatherhood. It is a journey that requires embracing emotions, seeking support, and ultimately finding peace in the new reality.

As Jim Stovall wisely stated, *"Life is not about what you have lost, but what you can still achieve."* This sentiment captures the essence of resilience and the ability to redefine one's path.

By embracing the lessons of individuals like Bethany Hamilton and Coach Robert Mendez Jr., fathers can find inspiration in their stories and strive to create a life filled with purpose and impact.

In the face of grief, remember that the journey of fatherhood is about building connections, celebrating achievements, and creating a legacy of love and support for your child. Embrace the challenges, honor your emotions, and find peace in the beautiful complexities of your family's journey. Through resilience and unwavering commitment, you can navigate the landscape of fatherhood with grace and strength, celebrating the unique gifts that your child brings to your life.

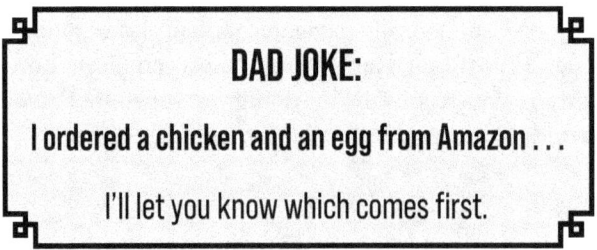

- 4 -
Being Present: Physically, Emotionally, and Spiritually for Your Child

I'M HERE FOR YOU

I stand beside you, hand in hand,
No need for words to understand.
The world may rush, the world may stare,
But here, right now, I'm fully there.

Not fixing, forcing, or asking why,
Just walking with you, step by stride.
Your laughter sings, your strength shines through,
And every moment, I learn from you.

At a minimum, society expects dads to provide financially. Each state has an agency or division that helps enforce child support orders. Skip making a child support payment and the state can garnish your wages or prevent you from renewing your driver's license. These punitive tactics are a source of family discord. At least the child support enforcement agencies have stopped chasing after "deadbeat dads," recognizing that some dads are simply dead broke.

Parenthood is a lifelong commitment, but when raising a child with special needs, the role of a father often takes on even greater significance. Your child may require more time, attention, and energy than you ever anticipated, and your presence—physically, emotionally, and spiritually—is a cornerstone of their growth and well-being. Yet being present isn't just about showing up. It involves engaging on multiple levels, understanding your child's needs deeply, and making intentional efforts to connect with them in ways that foster a sense of security, love, and belonging.

In this chapter, we'll explore what it means to truly be present for your child. Whether it's through active involvement in their day-to-day life, supporting them emotionally during challenging times, or guiding them spiritually, your presence is a gift that can empower your child and strengthen your bond. We'll discuss the importance of each of these aspects of presence and provide practical strategies to help you stay engaged with your child—no matter the demands or challenges of daily life.

The Power of Physical Presence

For most children, a father's physical presence represents safety, comfort, and reliability. Children with disabilities or special needs often rely even more heavily on the physical presence of their parents, as it provides consistency in a world that can feel overwhelming and unpredictable. Being physically present means more than simply being in the same room—it's about actively participating in your child's life, engaging in activities, and providing care and attention in ways that show you are invested in their well-being.

1. Show Up and Stay Engaged

Being physically present for your child requires you to make time in your schedule for them. This can be difficult, especially when balancing work, caregiving responsibilities, and other aspects of family life. However, the time you spend with your child—whether during play, therapy, or simply sharing a meal—is invaluable. It helps your child feel seen and heard and reassures them that they are a priority in your life.

- **Make Time for Daily Interaction:** Carve out time each day to spend with each of your children, even if it's just ten or fifteen minutes of focused interaction. This can be as simple as reading a book, going for a walk, or playing a game. The key is to be fully present during that time, without distractions from work, phones, or other responsibilities.
- **Be Present During Key Moments:** There are moments in your child's life that will require your focused attention—medical appointments, school meetings, therapy sessions, plays, recitals, and special occasions. Make it a priority to be present during these times. Your involvement sends a powerful message to your child: You care about their progress, health, and success. How will your children remember your presence? Were you the dad that rarely missed being there? If your dad was not present when you were growing up, you know what that feels like. Don't be that dad.

2. Participate in Daily Care

For many fathers, participating in the daily caregiving routines of a child with special needs can feel daunting. The tasks may include everything from feeding, dressing, bathing, and toileting to administering medication and attending therapy sessions. However, your active involvement in these routines not only strengthens your bond with your child but also helps you better understand their needs and abilities.

- **Take Turns with Caregiving:** If you have a partner, make sure to share caregiving responsibilities. This ensures that both parents are equally involved in the child's life and gives you more opportunities to connect with your child through care.
- **Learn Your Child's Routine:** Become familiar with your child's daily routine, including any specific medical or therapeutic needs. This familiarity will allow you to be a reliable source of support, and it reinforces your commitment to their well-being.

3. Physical Touch and Connection

Physical presence also includes touch, which is a powerful way to communicate love, safety, and connection. For children with special needs, especially those who may have sensory sensitivities, physical touch can either be comforting or overwhelming. It's important to understand your child's preferences and respond to their cues accordingly.

- **Affection Through Touch:** Many children with special needs, especially those with autism or sensory processing disorder, may have specific preferences for physical contact. Some may enjoy hugs, while others may prefer a gentle pat on the back or holding hands. Pay attention to what makes your child comfortable and respect their boundaries. If you can, ask what they prefer.
- **Physical Play:** Engage in physical activities that your child enjoys, such as playing sports, swimming, or simply rolling around on the floor together. Physical play is not only a fun way to bond but also an opportunity to support your child's motor skills and physical development. **Dick Hoyt**, one of the most iconic dads I've ever met, tells some amazing stories about how he involved Rick (his oldest son, who was a spastic quadriplegic, unable to talk or walk) in virtually all the family's activities.

> *That night, Rick, using his computer, said, "Dad, when I'm out running, it feels like my disability disappears." That was very powerful—and it was just the beginning.*
>
> *Our message is: Yes, you can. You can do anything you want to do as long as you make up your mind. You can do it.*
>
> —**Dick Hoyt,** *Dad To Dad Podcast,* **episode #11**

4. Make Education a Priority

As mentioned in the introduction, if dads could do just one thing it would be to fully engage in their child's education. All the research supports that when both parents are involved in a child's education, educational outcomes increase dramatically. When the Parent Teacher Association was established in 1925, the PTA was composed of both dads and moms. Although the original framing was inclusive, in practice the leadership and volunteer base quickly became dominated by women. Scholars note that by the mid-twentieth century, PTA units across the US were overwhelmingly staffed and led by mothers and women community volunteers, reflecting broader gendered expectations for maternal involvement in schooling. One of the unintended consequences of that shift in leadership was to give dads a pass on being more actively involved in their children's education. While that might be a cultural phenomenon, the fact remains that when both parents are actively involved in their child's education, the kids do better and society at large benefits.

As it relates to education and disabilities, most parents are totally unprepared for the world of IEPs (Individualized Education Programs), which we will delve into in more detail in Chapter 12. Our role as fathers at the IEP table is of critical importance. Here are some action-oriented ideas for enhancing your educational involvement:

- **Assume Competence:** For good or bad, when many parents get a diagnosis, a well-meaning doctor or health-care professional might say to you, "Your son/daughter will never be able to (fill in the blank): walk, talk, see, hear, etc." With all due respect, only God knows what our children will be capable of doing.
- **Start Reading to Your Kids at a Young Age:** Research indicates the years birth to three are the most formative years for brain

development. Regardless of your child's diagnosis, be the parent who reads to your child. It's not a gender-specific skill.
- **Attend All the Parent-Teacher Meetings:** You're probably thinking, easier said than done. Be the dad that errs on the side of prioritizing these periodic meetings and especially the IEP meetings. You send a strong message to your child's teachers and those involved with the IEP process.
- **Know Your Child's Teachers by Name:** Be the dad who knows all your child's teachers by name. If you have more than one child, it may be helpful to keep a small address book with names, phone numbers, and email addresses. The teachers will appreciate your involvement, and you will send a very powerful message to your child that you're totally dialed into what's going on at school.
- **Review Your Child's Homework and Grade Reports:** Develop a firsthand understanding of your child's strengths and weaknesses. Encourage them to do their best. Celebrate their successes and share stories about subjects you struggled with as a youth.
- **Seek Out Tutors:** In today's time-strapped world seek out tutors who may be able to supplement the time required to assist your child to grasp the subject matter.

The Importance of Emotional Presence

While physical presence is vital, being emotionally present for your child is just as critical. Emotional presence means being attuned to your child's feelings, offering empathy and support, and creating an environment where they feel safe to express their emotions. Children with special needs may have difficulty processing or communicating their emotions, so your role as an emotionally present father is to help them navigate their feelings with patience, understanding, and love.

1. Active Listening and Emotional Validation

Children, especially those with special needs, may struggle to articulate their emotions. This can lead to frustration, meltdowns, or withdrawal. By being an emotionally available father, you help create a space where your child feels heard and understood.

- **Listen Without Judging:** When your child is upset or trying to communicate their feelings, listen without interrupting or jumping to conclusions. Sometimes, they may not have the words to

explain their emotions, but your willingness to listen is a powerful affirmation that their feelings matter.
- **Validate Their Emotions:** Whether your child is sad, angry, or overwhelmed, it's important to validate their emotions. Acknowledge their feelings by saying things like, "I understand you're feeling upset," or "It's okay to feel frustrated." This helps them feel seen and encourages emotional growth.
- **Offer Reassurance:** Children with special needs often feel anxious or uncertain in new or challenging situations. Offering reassurance through words, actions, and gentle touch can help them feel more secure. Let them know you are there for them, no matter what.

Rooster Rossiter, a retired career US Marine, discovered his daughter Ainsley, who was diagnosed with neuroaxonal dystrophy, a rare genetic disorder, loved the feeling of the wind in her hair. That, combined with Rooster's commitment to spend more time with her, propelled him to get a special running chair and start training and signing up for 5Ks, 10Ks, half- and eventually full marathons. They were able to enjoy eight years of training and racing before Ainsley died as a result of the disease at age 12. Perhaps most impressively and well before Ainsley passed away, Rooster cofounded Ainsley's Angels, an organization that has provided more than three thousand running/racing chairs to like-minded people being physically present through running.

I'm Kim "Rooster" Rossiter, cofounder and president of Ainsley's Angels of America—and perhaps most importantly, Ainsley's dad. It gives me a great opportunity to come together with this inspired family here in Baton Rouge, Louisiana.

One day, a physical therapist named Peggy said we should go down to the local oceanfront and allow Ainsley the chance to roll with the wind. We saw how the wind blew in Ainsley's face, and it lit her up. We saw how she reacted to that wonderful excitement of the crowd—telling her that yes, she can accomplish a 5K road race, despite the fact that she's never taken a step in her life.

It makes me feel empowered. I feel like I can do anything in the world.

—Rooster Rossiter, *Dad To Dad Podcast*, **episode #29**

2. Patience and Understanding in Difficult Moments

Emotional presence also means being patient and calm in moments of distress. Children with special needs can sometimes experience emotional outbursts or behavior that seems challenging, especially in response to sensory overload, frustration, or difficulty communicating. Your ability to remain calm, patient, and understanding in these moments will help your child feel supported and safe.

- **Stay Calm in Crisis:** During meltdowns or emotional outbursts, your child is looking to you for stability. By staying calm and composed, you provide a sense of security that can help de-escalate the situation. **Doug Noll** is author of the book *De-Escalate: How to Calm an Angry Person in 90 Seconds or Less*, which teaches practical, neuroscience-informed listening and communication techniques to quickly defuse anger and transform volatile interactions into calm, constructive engagement in 90 seconds or less. This book could be your lifeline to marital and family harmony.

> *Neuroscientists now understand that every single thing we do is emotional. You can't even be rational or engage in critical thinking unless you're emotional first. That's the big insight.*
>
> *The basic human premise is this: We want to be heard and understood. We have two foundational needs that are not met in modern culture. Number one, to be heard and validated at a very deep emotional level. And number two, the need to be emotionally safe.*
>
> —Doug Noll, *Dad To Dad Podcast*, episode #217

- **Model Emotional Regulation:** As a father, you are one of your child's primary role models for emotional regulation. By demonstrating how to manage your own emotions—whether it's stress, anger, or frustration—you teach your child valuable skills for managing their own feelings.
- **Encourage Healthy Coping Mechanisms:** Help your child develop coping strategies for managing their emotions. Whether it's taking deep breaths, practicing mindfulness, or using calming techniques, these strategies can help your child feel more in control of their emotions.

3. Building Emotional Resilience

Children with special needs often face more challenges than their peers, which can sometimes affect their self-esteem and emotional well-being. As a father, your emotional presence can help build your child's resilience, teaching them how to navigate life's challenges with confidence and self-assurance.

- **Celebrate Their Strengths:** One of the most powerful ways to build emotional resilience in your child is by celebrating their strengths and abilities. Focus on what they can do, rather than what they struggle with. This boosts their confidence and helps them see themselves in a positive light. It took **Nik Nikic** more than a decade to embrace the fact that his son, Chris, who has Down syndrome, was gifted in different ways than his older sister. Chris joined a local triathlon club, learned to ride a bike at age 16, and before he knew it, he graduated from the sprint distance to the Olympic distance, then the half Ironman and eventually the full Ironman distance. In fact, Chris is the first person in the world with Down syndrome to complete the Ironman distance triathlon. Interestingly, I was present when Chris completed the Florida Ironman in November 2020, which was the second Ironman event in which I had competed. My handicap was that I turned 60 the month before.

One of the biggest lessons I learned as I started to realize what was possible was this: I have two children—one is 30, and Chris is 20. I realized that for the first 18 years of Chris's life, I treated Chris differently than I treated Jackie. And the result was different.

One day, over the last year or so, it hit me. I asked myself, "If Chris were born a typical child, what would his life be like?" And I started thinking—well, he'd probably be about six-foot-eight or nine. He'd probably be playing college basketball. I would have him at the gym at six in the morning, training hard, right?

> *And all of a sudden, I started thinking: If that's what I would have done with him if he didn't have Down syndrome, then why am I not treating him the same way now? The same way I treated my daughter.*
>
> *I helped my daughter become a successful college basketball player. But I treated them differently. I treated her as gifted, and I treated him as special. And what that meant was we protected him more and did more for him—which actually enabled him to become less.*
>
> —Nik Nikic, *Dad To Dad Podcast*, episode #108

- **Encourage Perseverance:** When your child faces challenges, encourage them to keep trying, even when things feel difficult. Offer praise for their efforts, not just the outcomes. By teaching them to embrace challenges with resilience, you help them develop a growth mindset that will serve them well throughout life.

Frank McKinney is a real estate artist who has written nine best-selling books, survived cancer, and competed thirteen times in the Badwater 135, one of the world's most grueling ultramarathons, covering 135 miles from the scorching depths of Death Valley, California—often above 120°F—to the portal of Mount Whitney in California, in July each year. With over 14,000 feet of cumulative ascent, runners battle extreme heat, relentless climbs, and sleep deprivation. This race is widely regarded as the ultimate test of human endurance and mental toughness. One of Frank's mantras is the importance of relentless forward motion.

> *You need to go against the grain. You need to not be afraid to take risks in life.*
>
> *When we'd be in an airport and there was a moving sidewalk, David, I would have her walk down the opposite direction. Because that's how life is. It's always coming at you. It's always telling you, "You can't do this. Little girl, you're going to get hurt. Little girl, you're on the wrong side."*
>
> *That's life. Until one day she finally said, "Dad, I'm too old to do this." That's when I stopped having her walk the wrong way.*
>
> —Frank McKinney, *Dad To Dad Podcast*, episode #260

Spiritual Presence: Guiding Your Child's Heart

Spiritual presence refers to the ways in which you guide your child in their understanding of values, purpose, and the deeper meaning of life. Spirituality can take many forms, from religious beliefs to a sense of connection to something greater than oneself. For children with special needs, a father's spiritual presence can offer comfort, hope, and a sense of purpose, helping them feel grounded and supported as they navigate the complexities of their world.

Rabbi Bradley Artson, who is a professor of philosophy and dean at American Jewish University in Los Angeles, I think said it best:

> *I tell people that one of the blessings of having a son with autism is that I'm the only dad I know whose 25-year-old will give him a full-body hug.*
>
> *My love for Jacob was and is ferocious, and we enjoy each other's presence.*
>
> *I believe all people have the right to communicate, which means our job is to figure out how to gain access to their intention and their content.*
>
> *In the end, we were able to hold on to each other and create a family that really is at the very heart of my heart—and it keeps me going.*
>
> —**Rabbi Bradley Artson**, *Dad To Dad Podcast*, **episode #25**

1. Sharing Faith and Spiritual Values

If you have a particular faith or spiritual practice, sharing it with your child can be a powerful way to connect and instill a sense of purpose and belonging. Children with special needs may find comfort in the routines and rituals of spiritual practice, as well as in the sense of community that often accompanies it.

- **Incorporate Spiritual Rituals:** Whether it's through prayer, meditation, or attending religious services, incorporate spiritual rituals into your family's routine. Sometimes families can find it difficult to attend religious services because the faith community isn't accessible or accepting of their child's needs or behavior. Sometimes families have to search for a religious group that specifically serves people with special needs. But these spiritual rituals can provide your child with a sense of structure and belonging, while also offering a deeper connection to their spiritual life.

- **Teach Values Through Stories and Actions:** Use stories from your faith or spiritual tradition to teach important values like kindness, compassion, and resilience. These values are especially important for children with special needs, as they navigate a world that may sometimes feel unkind or difficult to understand.

Steve Bundy works for Joni and Friends, the global Christian disability ministry, and is coauthor of the book *Another Kind of Courage: God's Design for Fathers of Families Affected by Disability*. Steve has a lot to say about the strength gained from having a deep faith.

> *He's a bundle of blessing—but a bundle of challenge at the same time. I didn't know what to do with all the emotion going on inside me, which is one of the reasons I'm so excited for the Special Fathers Network....*
>
> *That there's hope. There's a future. Someone to say, "You know what? You've got this." Someone to bounce questions off. How do I guard my marriage in the midst of all these challenges?*
>
> —Steve Bundy, *Dad To Dad Podcast*, episode #34

2. Finding Meaning in Life's Challenges

Raising a child with special needs can sometimes feel overwhelming, and it's natural to question why certain challenges arise. Spiritual presence involves helping your child (and yourself) find meaning and purpose amid these challenges.

- **Discuss the Bigger Picture:** Depending on your child's developmental level, engage them in discussions about life's challenges and the bigger picture. Talk about how difficulties can help us grow, and how every person's journey is unique and valuable.
- **Offer Hope and Encouragement:** Spiritual presence is also about offering hope. Even in difficult moments, remind your child that they are loved, valued, and part of something greater. Your words of encouragement can help them see beyond their immediate struggles and focus on the possibilities that lie ahead.

Tim Kuck, whose son, Nathaniel, only lived to age four before succumbing to multiple birth anomalies including duodenal atresia and craniosynostosis, went on to cofound Nathaniel's Hope, an Orlando,

Florida, nonprofit whose mission is to celebrate kids with special needs (the VIPs) as well as educate and equip communities and churches about serving the special needs families. The annual MAKE 'm SMILE event hosted by Nathaniel's Hope is a vibrant, family-friendly festival that attracts more than six thousand attendees, which celebrates kids and adults with special needs with entertainment, games, food, resource exhibitors, and a friendship stroll.

> *Our story did not end with the happy ending that we might have wanted at the time. But it's a happy ending. Because one day there's going to be a great reunion in heaven. And it's by the grace of God that we were able to take our son's life and death and pull alongside and encourage others as they walk through their trials in life. And so though our son died, a lot earlier than we would have liked him to, we were privileged to have him for four and a half years. And we know that one day there'll be a grand reunion. So there is a happy ending.*
>
> —Tim Kuck, *Dad To Dad Podcast*, **episode #57**

3. Connecting with Nature and the World Around Them

For some children, spirituality is deeply connected to the natural world. Encourage your child to spend time in nature, as it can provide a sense of peace, wonder, and connection to something larger than themselves.

- **Explore Nature Together:** Whether it's a walk in the park, a visit to the beach, or simply spending time in the backyard, explore nature together. Nature can be a calming and grounding experience for children with special needs, helping them feel connected to the world around them.
- **Foster Curiosity and Awe:** Encourage your child's natural curiosity about the world. Whether it's through exploring nature, asking big questions about life, or engaging in creative activities, fostering a sense of wonder helps your child feel connected to something greater than themselves.

Conclusion: The Gift of Presence

Being present—financially, physically, emotionally, and spiritually—for your child is one of the most profound gifts you can offer. Your presence provides a foundation of love, security, and connection that will shape their development and well-being throughout their life. While the challenges of raising a child with special needs can sometimes feel overwhelming, remember that your presence, in all its forms, is a source of strength, not only for your child but for you as well.

As you continue this journey, know that the time and attention you give your child are invaluable. Your physical presence shows them that they are a priority in your life. Your emotional presence teaches them that they are loved and understood. And your spiritual presence helps them find meaning, purpose, and hope in their journey. Together, these aspects of presence create a bond that will guide and support your child as they navigate the world, confident in the knowledge that they are never alone.

21st Century Dads Foundation created a fatherhood self-assessment tool based on the importance of being present, which can be found in Appendix A or at https://21stcenturydads.org/other-resources/.

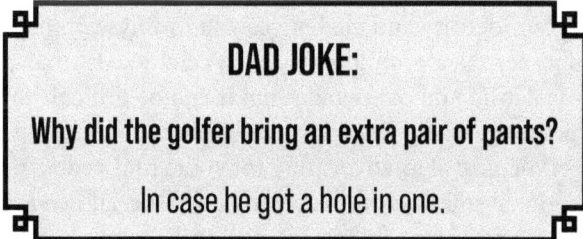

DAD JOKE:

Why did the golfer bring an extra pair of pants?

In case he got a hole in one.

- 5 -
Father-to-Father Mentoring: Wisdom, Support, and Strength in Community

BROTHERHOOD OF FATHERS

Through trials deep, we stand as one,
Fathers bound by love hard-won.
Guiding hands and open hearts,
Lifting each as strength imparts.

In whispered fears, in silent night,
We share the load, we share the light.
Raising children, bold and free,
Not defined by what they can't be.

Together we learn, together we grow,
Side by side, through highs and lows.
A brotherhood, steadfast and true,
For them, for us—we see it through.

Fatherhood is often described as a transformative journey, one that reshapes your identity and challenges you in ways you never expected. But for fathers raising children with special needs, that journey can feel uniquely isolating and overwhelming. It can be difficult to find others who truly understand your experiences—whether you're navigating the complexities of medical care, advocating for your child's education, or managing the emotional toll that often accompanies special needs parenting.

This is where father-to-father mentoring becomes invaluable. Connecting with other fathers who have walked a similar path offers not only emotional support but also practical wisdom and guidance that can make all the difference in your journey. Father-to-father mentoring provides a safe space for fathers to share their triumphs, struggles, fears, and hopes, fostering a sense of community and camaraderie that helps alleviate the sense of isolation many dads feel.

21st Century Dads Foundation's signature program is the **Special Fathers Network**, a dad-to-dad mentoring initiative specifically created for fathers raising children with special needs. Through this program, dads can connect with experienced mentors who understand the challenges of special needs parenting and can offer wisdom, support, and encouragement. In this chapter, we'll explore the power of father-to-father mentoring, and why it's such a critical resource for dads on this journey. We'll also dive into the impact of the Special Fathers Network and the ways in which mentoring helps fathers grow into stronger, more confident advocates for their children and families.

The Importance of Mentorship in Special Needs Parenting

Fatherhood, in any context, is filled with moments of uncertainty. But when you're raising a child with special needs, those uncertainties can multiply—each medical diagnosis, behavioral challenge, or developmental delay can leave you feeling unsure of what to do next. In these moments, mentorship from other fathers who have faced similar situations can be a lifeline. Mentorship not only provides practical advice but also offers emotional reassurance, reminding you that you are not alone on this journey.

1. Shared Experiences: The Power of Empathy

One of the most profound benefits of father-to-father mentoring is the power of shared experiences. When you connect with another dad who has walked a similar path, you are not just receiving advice—you are being seen and understood. That empathy is incredibly powerful. It's one thing to hear well-meaning advice from family members or friends, but when that advice comes from someone who has been in similar situations, it carries a different weight.

- **Understanding Without Explanation:** One of the challenges many fathers face is feeling the need to explain their child's condition or their family's situation to others. With father-to-father mentoring, often there's no need to explain. Your mentor has already been through similar experiences and understands the emotions and challenges that come with raising a child with special needs. This shared understanding fosters a deep sense of connection and reduces the feeling of isolation.

- **Empathy as a Bridge:** Empathy from another father builds trust and allows for honest, vulnerable conversations. Whether you're discussing your fears about your child's future, frustrations with the medical system, or concerns about maintaining balance in your marriage, your mentor can relate, offering validation and support.

Tony Oommen, a longtime friend, was the very first dad to share his story on the *SFN Dad To Dad Podcast*. Hearing other dads talk openly and authentically about their circumstances opens the door for others to do the same.

Imagine this. You're happily married. You have two children. And then…this happens.

I remember it like it was yesterday, when this all started. I had taken the kids to drive somewhere to buy my wife flowers for Valentine's Day. We were pulling back into our house. My son was six—still in a car seat. He had fallen asleep.

I was taking him out of his car seat when he suddenly went into a seizure. I had never seen one before, and it scared me to death. After that, he was non-responsive. He was breathing, but he wasn't responsive after that first seizure. I didn't know what was happening.

So I called my sister, who is a physician. She was engaged to someone who is an emergency room physician. I got on the phone with her then-fiancé, Matt, and he said, "You need to take him to the hospital."

He was rushed to the hospital. He had a series of seizures—over a hundred of them—during the five weeks he was hospitalized. What it turned out to be was a viral infection. The virus had crossed the blood-brain barrier into the central nervous system. And the brain and central nervous system don't have a defense mechanism against a virus.

Ben, fortunately, lived. But he came away with damage to his brain from that virus.

—**Tony Oommen**, *Dad To Dad Podcast*, **episode #1**

2. Practical Wisdom and Guidance

In addition to empathy, father-to-father mentoring provides practical wisdom that can make navigating special needs parenting more manageable. A mentor who has already gone through similar challenges can offer advice on everything from advocating for your child's educational needs to managing the day-to-day logistics of caregiving. This practical wisdom can be invaluable, especially for fathers who are just beginning their journey. **Randy Lewis**, who is a good friend and neighbor, is a former executive vice president at Walgreens. Randy has been a pioneer in the field of providing employment to people with all types of disabilities. Randy's lived experience, with his autistic son, Austin, combined with his leadership role, and his good sense of humor has been a beacon of hope for a wide range of dads.

> *Only 58 percent of young adults with autism are employed, and even fewer get married. I learned that disabilities play no favorites—rich, poor, Black, white, whatever color. Disabilities play no favorites.*
>
> *I was thinking about all those people—wealthy people, not-so-wealthy people—who struggle. What are they going to do? And here I am, in charge of this division. I've got ten thousand people and a billion-dollar budget. If I can't do something about this, who will?*
>
> *We're a successful company like Walgreens. And if Walgreens couldn't do something about it, which company would?*
>
> —Randy Lewis, *Dad To Dad Podcast*, episode #2

- **Navigating the Health-Care System:** The health-care system can feel like a maze when you're dealing with a child who has complex medical needs. While mentor fathers don't offer medical or legal advice (that's what doctors and lawyers do), they are uniquely qualified to offer well-informed insights based on their firsthand experiences. They can offer guidance on finding the right specialists, advocating for treatments, and managing medical paperwork. Their experience can save you time, energy, and stress.
- **Advocating for Educational Services:** Education is often one of the biggest challenges for parents of children with special needs. Whether it's navigating Individualized Education Programs

(IEPs), advocating for inclusion in general education classrooms, or finding the right school, your mentor can share strategies that have worked for their child. This guidance can empower you to become a stronger advocate for your own child's educational needs.

Catherine Whitcher is one of the most knowledgeable people on the planet when it comes to all things IEP. In fact, Catherine hosts her own podcast entitled *The Inner Circle Podcast*, which is an extraordinary resource for dads, moms, and caregivers.

This is kind of exciting—we get to share a story of hope, a story of success, and a story of possibilities.

That's a big part of what I share when I talk about my daughter. It's like, yes, we came from this dark place. But our journey was our journey. So many times in the special needs world, someone with a specific diagnosis looks to other families and assumes that's going to be their path. And it's not necessarily going to be that way.

—Catherine Whitcher, *Dad To Dad Podcast*, episode #202

- **Balancing Work and Family Life:** Many fathers struggle to balance their work responsibilities with the demands of caregiving. A mentor who has faced similar challenges can offer practical tips for time management, setting boundaries at work, and prioritizing self-care.

3. Emotional Support: Strengthening Resilience

The emotional toll of raising a child with special needs can be significant, and it's something that fathers often struggle to discuss openly. In many cases, societal expectations of fatherhood create an additional layer of pressure, with dads feeling like they must be the stoic providers who can't show vulnerability. Father-to-father mentoring offers a safe space for emotional expression, allowing fathers to process their feelings and build emotional resilience.

- **A Safe Space for Vulnerability:** One of the greatest gifts a mentor can offer is a safe space to be vulnerable. In many cases, fathers feel like they need to put on a brave face for their family, but that can lead to emotional burnout. Talking to another father who

understands the emotional challenges of special needs parenting can be incredibly cathartic. It allows fathers to express their fears, frustrations, and hopes without fear of judgment.
- **Building Emotional Resilience:** Emotional resilience is the ability to bounce back from challenges and continue moving forward, even when things feel overwhelming. Father-to-father mentoring helps build this resilience by offering support and encouragement during difficult times. Knowing that someone else has faced similar challenges and has come out stronger on the other side can be incredibly motivating.

4. Learning from the Journey: A Long-Term Perspective

Another benefit of father-to-father mentoring is the opportunity to gain a long-term perspective on your journey as a father. Often, when you're in the midst of a particularly difficult time—whether you're managing your child's health, dealing with behavioral issues, or navigating school systems—it's easy to feel like the struggle will never end. Talking to a mentor who has already traveled that road can offer hope and reassurance that, over time, things can improve, and you will continue to grow in your role as a father.

- **Hindsight and Growth:** Mentors who are further along in their journey can offer insights into the ways they've grown as fathers and the lessons they've learned. They can share stories of their own struggles and how they overcame them, offering a sense of perspective that can be reassuring to newer fathers.
- **Hope for the Future:** One of the greatest gifts a mentor can offer is hope. Hearing stories of other fathers who have successfully navigated the challenges of raising a child with special needs can help you feel more confident in your ability to handle whatever comes next.

The Special Fathers Network: Connecting Fathers to One Another

The **Special Fathers Network** is one of the most powerful examples of a father-to-father mentoring program designed specifically for dads raising children with special needs. The network was created in 2017 with the understanding that fathers can benefit from a supportive community of peers who can relate to their experiences. SFN provides a structured platform for fathers to connect with mentors who offer both emotional support and practical guidance.

1. What is the Special Fathers Network?

The Special Fathers Network is a growing community of fathers who are raising, or have raised, children with special health-care needs or disabilities. The program matches experienced fathers (mentor fathers) with dads who are closer to the beginning of their special needs parenting journey. These mentors provide one-on-one support, offering advice, encouragement, and resources to help newer fathers navigate the unique challenges of special needs parenting.

- **Personalized Mentoring:** The SFN pairs fathers based on their specific circumstances, ensuring that mentors have experience relevant to the mentee's needs. Whether you're raising a child with autism, Down syndrome, cerebral palsy, or a rare disease, the network can connect you with a mentor who understands your unique challenges.
- **A Global Community:** With fathers participating from around the world, the Special Fathers Network offers a diverse and rich community of experiences. This global reach means that fathers can connect with others who have similar experiences, even if they're living halfway across the world.

2. How the Special Fathers Network Helps Fathers Grow

One of the greatest strengths of the Special Fathers Network is its ability to foster growth in both mentors and mentees. While the primary goal is to support newer fathers, mentors often report that the process of mentoring others helps them reflect on their own journey and grow as fathers.

- **A Two-Way Street:** Mentoring is a two-way street, and mentors often find that they learn as much from their mentees as the mentees do from them. The process of sharing their experiences helps mentors gain new insights into their own parenting journey, and it reinforces the lessons they've learned along the way. Some of our most active SFN Mentor Fathers are in their 60s and 70s. They realize how important having these relationships can be. Virtually all these seasoned dads have said, "I wish there was a network like this when I was a younger dad." Some would further add, "I wasted so much time and energy trying to figure out everything myself and inadvertently isolating myself." Here are some testimonials from some of the more seasoned SFN Mentor Fathers, including **Rich Gathro** of Danville, Kentucky; **John Shouse** of Franklin, Tennessee; and **Jordan Jankus** of Wallingford, Vermont.

> *The Dad in the Middle experience allows us to raise questions to other dads whom we trust and have come to love. That's been valuable for me to raise my life questions with them, but it's also been because we fall in love with each other as brothers.*
>
> —Rich Gathro, *Dad To Dad Podcast*, episode #308

> *This is an investment in becoming a better father, becoming a better spouse, and becoming a better man. And if that's not worth at least $50—even in a tight budget—I don't know what is.*
>
> —John Shouse, *Dad To Dad Podcast*, episode #314

> *I had the absolute honor of being an advocate for her in life, because she can't advocate for herself in many ways.*
>
> *I appreciate the Mastermind Group because it makes the continuation of advocacy possible for me—even at my advanced age. It's nice to hear that other people are going through the same thing.*
>
> —Jordan Jankus, *Dad To Dad Podcast*, episode #330

- **Building Confidence:** For newer fathers, the support and guidance of a mentor can be transformative. It helps build confidence in their ability to handle the challenges of special needs parenting, and it offers reassurance that they are not alone in their journey. Some of the younger SFN dads claim the SFN has transformed their lives, including **Ian Todd** from Baltimore, Maryland, and **Joe Lofino** of Greenville, Ohio.

> *It's a great forum for me to help to get that off my chest. And it's also great to get the feedback from a lot of other people. Sometimes I just need a place to rant. Sometimes I honestly just need a place to be sad and for people to understand and what it feels like to have loss.*
>
> —Ian Todd, *Dad To Dad Podcast*, episode #320

> *It's changed my life drastically. I don't know if we would have had our third child because Fragile X is a genetic thing, so it was kind of risky. And I should mention all three of our kids, full mutation Fragile X.*
>
> —Joe Lofino, *Dad To Dad Podcast*, episode #336

3. The Role of Mentoring in Building Stronger Families

The Special Fathers Network doesn't just benefit the fathers who participate; the network also strengthens families. By providing fathers with the support they need, the network helps create a more balanced, supportive family dynamic.

- **Supporting Marriages:** One of the biggest challenges for families raising children with special needs is maintaining a strong marriage amid the stresses of caregiving. Father-to-father mentoring offers emotional support and practical advice that can help fathers navigate these challenges and maintain a healthy relationship with their partner.

Todd Evans of Brentwood, Tennessee, along with his wife, Kristin, coauthored the book *How to Build a Thriving Marriage as You Are Raising Children with Disabilities*, which offers practical advice on strengthening your marriage while meeting the demands of parenting.

> *If you see it as an investment in other dads, that's the way to look at it—an opportunity to help the organization and help set things up for other dads.*
>
> *For me, that's where the value is. Yes, there are benefits—like assistance with the retreat and tangible things that come back to me—but thinking of it as an investment in other dads really helps my mindset.*
>
> —**Todd Evans**, *Dad To Dad Podcast*, **episode #344**

- **Creating Stronger Bonds with Children:** When fathers feel more confident and supported in their role, they are better able to connect with their children. The insights and advice gained through strong mentoring can help fathers build stronger, more meaningful relationships with their children. One of Israel's most revered fathers is SFN Mentor Father **Doron Almog**, a retired major general in the Israel Defense Forces and founder of Aleh Negev (now known as Adi Negev-Nahalat Eran), a $50 million state-of-the-art residential and outpatient center serving Jews, Muslims, and Christians with disabilities and staffed by Jews, Muslims, and Christians. Doron credits his nonverbal autistic son, Eran, who passed away at age 23, with being his greatest teacher.

> *Despite the sadness and tragedy—and the burden and the suffering—understand that this is a huge test. And in this test, I think the highest value we must commit to is love.*
>
> *Loving your child. Loving your child with a disability.*
>
> —**Doron Almog**, *Dad To Dad Podcast*, **episode #100**

Conclusion: The Lifelong Impact of Mentorship

Father-to-father mentoring is a powerful tool for personal growth, emotional support, and practical wisdom. It fosters a sense of community among fathers, reminding them that they are not alone in their journey of raising a child with special needs. Programs like the Special Fathers Network play a crucial role in connecting dads across the globe, offering support that strengthens individual fathers and entire families.

By engaging in father-to-father mentoring, you're not just receiving help, you're becoming part of a community that celebrates the unique joys and challenges of special needs parenting. You're building lifelong friendships, gaining invaluable knowledge, and most importantly, finding strength in the shared journey. Through this support system, you'll be empowered to navigate the path ahead with greater confidence, resilience, and hope.

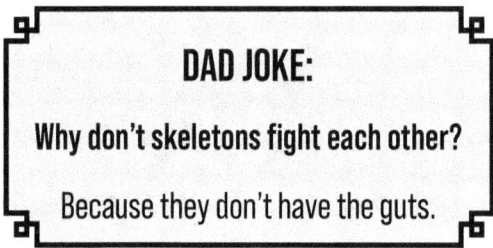

DAD JOKE:

Why don't skeletons fight each other?

Because they don't have the guts.

- 6 -
Self-Care for Dads: Prioritizing Your Well-Being to Better Serve Your Family

BEING SELFISH & SELFLESS

I dreamed of ease, a life so grand,
A path well-paved, a future planned.
Then you arrived, my heart stood still,
Not what I wished—but what was real.

I mourned my ease, my fleeting time,
The weight of care, the uphill climb.
But in your eyes, so pure, so bright,
I found my strength, I found my light.

Selfish first, but not for long,
Love redefined what makes me strong.
For in your world, so vast, so free,
I learned to give—wholeheartedly.

As a father raising a child with special needs, you've probably heard the saying, "You can't pour from an empty cup." While the demands of fatherhood are often overwhelming, this expression holds even more true for dads of children with special needs and disabilities. The unique challenges you face—navigating health-care systems, advocating for educational services, managing family dynamics—can easily leave you emotionally and physically drained. Yet, too often, fathers overlook their own well-being in the name of service to their families.

But the reality is this: Prioritizing your self-care is not a selfish act. It is essential for your long-term ability to be the present, supportive, and resilient father your child needs. In fact, the better you take care of yourself, the better you'll be able to care for your family. This chapter will explore why self-care is critical for fathers of children with special needs and provide practical strategies for integrating it into your daily life.

While it's honorable for parents to make their kids a priority and to be selfless, the truth is, you are not able to be selfless without first being selfish. Yes, you read that correctly. The only way to bring your A game consistently is to be selfish and that starts with self-care. **Rob Gorski**, the father of three autistic sons who is also known as the "Autism Dad," says it best.

> *What happened with Liz was she suffered from caretaker burnout. That's where you sort of give so much of yourself that there's literally nothing left to give. Just shut down. We ended up going through a separation for about two years. I had everything, the kids, on my own, while she lived with her parents.*
>
> *It took two years for her to get back on her feet. We now realize that we have to prioritize ourselves. You have to be selfish before you can be selfless.*
>
> —**Rob Gorski**, *Dad To Dad Podcast*, **episode #16**

The Myth of the Self-Sacrificing Father

For many men, societal expectations of fatherhood center around being a financial provider. The image of the self-sacrificing father who works long hours and forgoes personal pleasures for the sake of his family is pervasive. While these ideals come from a place of love and responsibility, they can lead to burnout, stress, resentment, and even health problems when taken to the extreme.

As a father of a child with special needs, the pressure to be "everything" for your family can feel even greater. Not only are you managing the typical responsibilities of fatherhood, but you're also navigating complex medical decisions, advocating for services, and emotionally supporting your child through their challenges. In this context, it's easy to believe that taking time for yourself is an indulgence you simply can't afford. But this mindset is unsustainable.

When fathers neglect their own needs, they eventually reach a breaking point. Physical exhaustion, emotional burnout, and mental health struggles can creep in, making it harder to be the dad your child and family need. By understanding the importance of self-care and making it a priority, you can maintain the strength, resilience, and balance necessary to navigate the challenges of special needs parenting.

The Importance of Self-Care for Fathers

At its core, self-care is about ensuring that your basic physical, emotional, and mental health needs are met. For fathers raising children with special needs, this often means taking steps to avoid burnout, manage stress, and recharge your emotional batteries. By prioritizing self-care, you're not just taking care of yourself; you're creating the foundation for a healthier, more balanced family life.

Dr. Judson Brandeis, a board-certified urologist and author of the book *21st Century Man: Advice from 50 Top Doctors and Men's Health Experts So You Can Feel Great, Look Good and Have Better Sex*, has created one of the most comprehensive resources for men's health and well-being. Consider getting yourself a copy of the book. The price of the book is a small investment that will pay a lifetime of benefits.

> *One of the great things about my medical practice is my patients. They're just fantastic—really hardworking, good guys.*
>
> *I think guys have taken a real beating over the past five or ten years because of people like Weinstein and Epstein. But 99 percent of the guys out there are really good people. They work hard, take care of their families, take care of their jobs, and take care of their communities. They don't expect other people to take care of them.*
>
> *At the same time, it's really important to understand that you **do** have to take care of yourself. And if you don't take care of yourself, you can't take care of other people.*
>
> —Dr. Judson Brandeis, *Dad To Dad Podcast*, episode #228

1. Managing Stress

Stress is an inevitable part of parenting. Whether it's dealing with unexpected medical emergencies, advocating for your child's rights, or simply managing the day-to-day challenges of caregiving, the stressors can quickly pile up. Without healthy outlets for managing this stress, it can lead to physical symptoms like headaches, fatigue, and insomnia, as well as emotional symptoms like anxiety, irritability, resentment, and depression.

By incorporating self-care practices into your routine, you can manage stress more effectively. Simple activities like exercise, meditation, or even taking a few moments of quiet reflection can help reduce stress levels and prevent burnout. The key is consistency—making self-care a regular part of your life, rather than something you only turn to in moments of crisis.

- **Exercise as a Stress Reliever:** Physical activity is one of the most effective ways to reduce stress. Whether it's going for a run, hitting the gym, or practicing yoga, exercise releases endorphins, which naturally boost your mood and help you feel more energized. Even just twenty to thirty minutes of exercise a day can have a significant impact on your mental and emotional well-being.

Adam Levy is a personal fitness trainer. One of his superpowers and one of the keys to his success in overcoming the challenges of having a young daughter with complex medical needs is maintaining his physical fitness and showing others how to do the same.

In the morning and afternoons, I was personal training, because I really needed some human connection. I also needed some control over the outcome of my effort, and I found training to have its value, but also it did not provide me an outlet for exerting myself on the world and seeing the impact there.

—**Adam Levy,** *Dad To Dad Podcast*, **episode #22**

- **Mindfulness and Meditation:** Mindfulness practices, such as meditation or deep breathing exercises, can help you manage stress by keeping you grounded in the present moment. These techniques teach you to focus on your breath, quiet your mind, and release tension, which can be particularly helpful during moments of being overwhelmed.

Azim Khamisa lost his only son, Tariq, in 1995 at age 20 to a violent crime. The grief and sense of loss were crippling. Azim credits his commitment to mindfulness and meditation to providing him with a way forward. In his book *The Secrets of a Bulletproof Spirit: How to Bounce Back from Life's Hardest Hits*, Azim outlines how you can also embrace mindfulness and meditation.

> *And I teach in one of my books that a healthy way to grieve is to journal. Spend time with nature, meditate, pray, read something inspiring. I spent some time with family and close friends, but did not have a social life during that time. I wrote my first book* From Murder to Forgiveness, *which was three years after Tariq died.*
>
> —Azim Khamisa, *Dad To Dad Podcast*, **episode #147**

2. Emotional Resilience

Emotional resilience, the ability to bounce back from challenges, is essential for fathers raising children with special needs. Without it, the emotional toll of caregiving can leave you feeling depleted, anxious, and disconnected. Self-care practices that nurture your emotional well-being, such as connecting with a supportive community or engaging in hobbies you enjoy, help build this resilience.

- **Connecting with Other Fathers:** One of the most powerful ways to build emotional resilience is by connecting with other fathers who understand your experiences. This could be through a support group, an online community, or a father-to-father mentoring program like the Special Fathers Network. By sharing your challenges and triumphs with other dads, you gain emotional support, perspective, and encouragement that can help sustain you through difficult times.
- **Hobbies and Creative Outlets:** Engaging in hobbies or creative activities that bring you joy can be an excellent form of self-care. Whether it's playing music, painting, gardening, or woodworking, these activities offer an opportunity to relax, express yourself, and recharge emotionally. By carving out time for activities you enjoy, you're giving yourself permission to step away from the demands of caregiving.

Scott Newport of Royal Oak, Michigan, lost his son, Evan, at age seven to Noonan syndrome, a rare genetic disease. A former carpenter, Scott has combined his woodworking skills and commitment to support families touched by disability. Scott utilizes discarded and damaged wood to create useful devices and gives them as gifts to families struggling with loss.

I had just finished building a staircase, and there was one tread in the staircase that had a knot in it, and I thought the customer would never accept it. It was kind of a damaged piece of junk. So I took that step, and I cut the top out of it, and I had some other scrap pieces I actually had in my garbage can. I pulled those out, and I was able to make four legs and a top. And I thought, "Oh, this is pretty cool. He'll never know that it was out of the garbage." So I took it to the hospital.

About a week later, I had it all finished, and I said, "Hey, Doctor Bob," or whoever it was, "Can we talk? I made you something."

And as I was presenting it to him, I started to think about my son, Evan, right? He had a heart defect. He had Noonan syndrome. Kind of like a throwaway, right? Nobody wants a kid like that. And I started to cry, and he started to cry. And that's where it all started, where I started finding the beauty in the brokenness, right? And especially our kids with special health-care needs and disabilities.

—**Scott Newport**, *Dad To Dad Podcast*, **episode #179**

3. Physical Health and Well-Being

Your physical health is the foundation of your ability to care for your family. Yet, for many fathers, physical self-care often falls to the bottom of the priority list. Long hours at work, sleepless nights, and the constant demands of parenting can make it easy to neglect things like proper nutrition, sleep, and regular medical check-ups. However, neglecting your physical health can lead to burnout, fatigue, and even serious health problems down the line.

- **Prioritizing Sleep:** Sleep is one of the most critical aspects of self-care, yet it's often the first thing to be sacrificed when life gets busy. As a father of a child with special needs, you may find yourself waking up in the middle of the night to care for your child or worrying about their future. However, chronic sleep deprivation can have serious consequences for both your physical and mental health. The rule of thumb is to get at least seven to eight hours of sleep a night, and if you're struggling with insomnia or disrupted sleep, consider talking to a health-care professional for support.

To be totally transparent, I've been fortunate to need much less sleep than average. When I was younger, I could get by on five hours per night, and I very rarely (about once a year) use an alarm to wake up. Now at age 65 and enlightened about the importance of and healing power of sleep, I am more mindful about the amount of sleep and type of sleep I'm getting. To be more intentional, I use a Fitbit to track my sleep. Whether it's a Fitbit, Apple Watch, Garmin, or some other device, do yourself a favor and be more intentional about the amount and quality of your sleep.

- **Eating Well:** Proper nutrition is another cornerstone of physical self-care. Eating a balanced diet that includes plenty of fruits, vegetables, lean proteins, and whole grains can help you maintain your energy levels and support your overall health. It can be tempting to rely on convenience foods when life feels overwhelming, but investing time in consuming healthy meals can make a big difference in how you feel.
- **Family Meal Rituals:** Eating meals together as a family with consistency is also one of the key factors to maintaining a healthy family life. While this becomes increasingly difficult as children get older and are involved in activities, the ritual of having dinners together has been documented to improve nutrition, create stronger family bonds, reduce the chances of high-risk behaviors in children, as well as positive impacts on mental and academic performance. Yes, you read that correctly: improved academic performance. For more information go to thefamilydinnerproject.org.

4. Mental Health and Professional Support

News Alert, Beware of Testosterone Poisoning! Fundamental fact: We're the gender that doesn't pull over and ask for directions when we're lost. While there are many positive aspects of staying on task and not giving up, the enlightened father will know when to seek advice. It's not a weakness but rather a strength to ask for help. While many fathers hesitate to seek professional help for mental health concerns, it's important to recognize that therapy, counseling, or even life coaching can be powerful tools for self-care. Raising a child with special needs comes with unique emotional challenges, and it's okay to ask for help when you need it.

- **Therapy and Counseling:** Talking to a therapist or counselor can provide you with a safe space to process your emotions, develop coping strategies, and work through any feelings of stress, anxiety, or depression you may be experiencing. Therapy is not a sign of weakness—it's a proactive step toward maintaining your emotional well-being.

- **Life Coaching and Personal Development:** For fathers looking to improve their personal growth, life coaching can be a valuable resource. Life coaches can help you set goals, manage your time more effectively, and find ways to balance your responsibilities with your personal aspirations. This type of support can be especially helpful for fathers who feel stuck or overwhelmed in their current situation.

Riana Milne of Del Ray Beach, Florida, is a licensed mental health counselor, a global life and love coach, and a best-selling author. Riana says it best:

The difference between therapy and coaching is that in therapy, most people call you a patient, which connotes you're sick. I always call my therapy clients "clients." We're there together working on an issue or a problem. So, I'm very solution focused, motivational, inspirational. What can we do? Not focus on the negative, the fears, and what we can't do, right? So, I always had a very different style from therapists from day one.

—Riana Milne, *Dad To Dad Podcast*, episode #203

Practical Self-Care Strategies for Dads

Now that we've explored the importance of self-care, let's dive into some practical strategies you can use to integrate self-care into your daily life. While every father's situation is different, these strategies can be adapted to fit your unique needs and circumstances.

1. Create a Daily Self-Care Routine

One of the most effective ways to prioritize self-care is to create a daily routine that incorporates activities that nurture your physical, emotional, and mental health. This routine doesn't have to be complicated or time-consuming; it could be as simple as setting aside ten minutes in the morning for meditation, going for a short walk during your lunch break, or spending fifteen minutes journaling before bed.

Warren Rustand of Tucson, Arizona, is one of the most intentional and well-respected people I've ever met. Warren is the author of *The Leader Within Us: Mindset, Principles, and Tools for a Life by Design* and recognized leader within the YPO (Young Presidents' Organization), the WPO (World Presidents' Organization), and the EO (Entrepreneurs' Organization). One of his daily rituals is his 10-10-10-1 rule.

> *Sit on the edge of your bed. Ask yourself, why are you alive today? What's my purpose today? Then spend ten minutes in gratefulness. Think of all the things in your life that you can be grateful for. And then spend ten minutes reading inspiration, positive inspiration. And then spend ten minutes positively journaling for the next generation.*
>
> *And leave those journals for your children and grandchildren to absorb. Don't write about the bad stuff. Write about the good stuff. You can write about the good lessons that you learned from bad stuff. But write about the good stuff.*
>
> *Now you're thirty-one minutes into your day. A minute of deciding your purpose, ten minutes of a gratefulness, ten minutes of inspirational reading, ten minutes of journaling. You have to ask yourself, where is your mind? It's ready to go. You're in a positive frame of mind.*
>
> —Warren Rustand, *Dad To Dad Podcast*, **episode #142**

- **Morning Routine:** Start your day with intention by creating a morning routine that sets a positive tone for the day ahead. This could include working out, going for a run, simply stretching, drinking a glass of water, practicing gratitude, or setting a positive affirmation for the day. Early in my career, I learned some valuable lessons from cold-calling. Yes, I was one of "those people." As young financial advisors we were expected to make at least one hundred outgoing calls a day. If you do the math, that's five hundred per week, two thousand per month and twenty-four thousand per year. You had to be a glutton for punishment, putting up with 99 percent rejection of one type or another. It was an exercise in humility and taught me so many lessons. It teaches you not to take rejection personally, i.e., don't let what people say, think, or do hurt your feelings. Another lesson was doing the hard things first

(cold-calling) every morning, before the demands of the workday/daily life start to pile up.
- **Midday Breaks:** If possible, schedule short breaks throughout your day to recharge. This could be as simple as stepping outside for fresh air, doing a brief breathing exercise, or enjoying a healthy snack.
- **Evening Wind-Down:** End your day with activities that help you relax and unwind. This might include reading a book, spending time with your partner, or practicing mindfulness. One daily habit I picked up because of going through the Catholic Church's RICA (Right of Christian Initiation for Adults) back in 2011 was to create a gratitude journal. Up until that point I thought journaling was something only teenage girls did. Every night before going to bed I record five to eight things I'm thankful for. At first it was a stretch to come up with just a few. Over time and with some training, it helps you focus on some important and positive things that take place every day. By doing this before going to bed, you're programming your subconscious to take over on a positive note as you fall asleep. One other thing about evening routines: No electronic devices or screens thirty minutes before going to sleep, and for goodness' sake, don't keep your phone on the nightstand.

2. Set Boundaries and Compartmentalize.

As a father, you may feel pressure to be constantly available to your family, work, and other responsibilities. However, setting boundaries is an essential part of self-care. Learn to say "no" to activities or commitments that drain your energy or take time away from your self-care. By setting clear boundaries, you're creating space for the activities that truly matter and protecting your own well-being.

- **Work-Life Balance:** If your job is demanding, like mine was when our kids were young, it's important to set boundaries around your work hours. I think of it as compartmentalizing. One of the decisions that helped me navigate ten-hour workdays was to get up super early, work out, and catch the 5:07 a.m. train into the city. Doing so allowed me to be home by 5:30 p.m., in time for dinner and after-dinner routines with the family.
- Since the COVID-19 pandemic and with so many people working remotely now, the idea of compartmentalizing is even more important. Some dads have created a separate workspace with a

door. When the door is open, the kids know dad is available, and when it's shut, everyone knows "Daddy is at work" and should not be interrupted. Obviously that approach takes some getting used to and extra discipline on everyone's part.
- The workplace is evolving and changing. For those who are not self-employed, communicate with your employer about your family's needs and find ways to balance your professional responsibilities with your role as a father.
- Some special needs dads have decided to change careers to jobs that are more flexible and less demanding schedule-wise. Take **Jeff Johnson** in Anderson, South Carolina. More than a decade ago, Jeff traded his management job at Publix for the role of a meat cutter, to spend more time with and help care for his son, Daniel, who is now 27 years old, nonverbal, and unable to walk, feed, or bathe himself.

> *To see deliberate movement in his eyes—to make something happen on that computer screen—I'll be honest with you, I wasn't sure it was going to work. And shame on me for not having more faith in Daniel.*
>
> *To sit there and watch him activate that computer—not as a random act, but something he was intentionally doing—was absolutely incredible. And of course, the tears came again—tears of joy, happiness, and excitement.*
>
> —**Jeff Johnson**, *Dad To Dad Podcast*, **episode #155**

- **Protecting Personal Time:** As stated previously, we need to be selfish, before we can be selfless. I'm a firm believer in compartmentalizing. Focus on work during work hours, focus on family during family time, and focus on ourselves during our personal time. What interests or hobbies do you have that provide you with some level of personal satisfaction? This might range from watching your favorite sports team, to reading or listening to an educational or inspirational book or podcast, to training for a 10K race, a half-marathon, or triathlon. **Jeff Johnson**, mentioned above, and his wife, Michelle, find time to run on a weekly basis and advocate for others through Ainsley's Angels.
- **Be Intentional, but Flexible:** The most important aspect is being intentional. While parenting can be challenging and

unpredictable, those who have a plan, budget for it, develop a routine, and follow through are much more likely to have better and healthier outcomes.
- **Reciprocity:** Let's face an important truth: Most of us dads are not "solo" parents, i.e., no mom in the picture at all. Whether you're still married or not, the mother of your children also needs to practice self-care. Helping her stay healthy and encouraging her to find ways to manage stress, be a healthy eater, and make time for herself is equally important. Keep in mind what works for you will likely be different from what works for your spouse. While it might be difficult to embrace at first, things like manicures, meeting with her book club, playing her favorite sport, and girls' nights out can make a real difference.

Conclusion: A Family's Cornerstone

When you make your physical, emotional, and spiritual well-being a priority, you are not taking time away from your family—you are strengthening your capacity to lead, love, and endure for the long journey ahead. A healthy father is not a luxury in a family raising a child with special needs; he is a cornerstone.

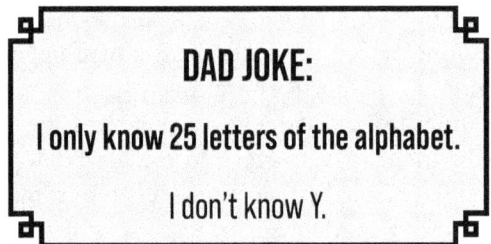

DAD JOKE:

I only know 25 letters of the alphabet.

I don't know Y.

-7-
Respite and Renewal: The Importance of Taking Breaks Without Guilt

STEADY HANDS, OPEN HEART

In weary nights and endless days,
I walk this path in love's embrace.
My child's light, so fierce, so bright,
Guides me through the darkest nights.

But strength must rest, a flame must breathe,
To give, I too must first receive.
A steady hand, a soul renewed,
So I can give my best to you.

In the journey of dads raising a child with special needs, the weight of responsibility can feel immense. As dads, we often share the role of caregivers, advocates, and sources of strength for our families. The emotional and physical demands can be overwhelming, leading many fathers (and mothers) to neglect their own need for rest and rejuvenation. Yet the truth is that taking breaks is not just beneficial; it's essential for our well-being and effectiveness as parents. This chapter will explore the importance of respite, strategies for finding time for yourself, and how to embrace breaks without guilt.

Understanding Respite: A Vital Component of Caregiving

Respite care is defined as short-term relief for primary caregivers, allowing them to take a break from their responsibilities. It can often be arranged through various means, including family members, friends, professional caregivers, or specialized respite care programs. For many families, finding respite can be very difficult—either finding someone willing and able to care for their child or paying for such care. For fathers of children with special needs, respite can provide a critical opportunity to recharge, regain perspective, and cultivate personal interests that often get sidelined.

The Necessity of Respite

The nature of caregiving can be all-consuming. While it is rewarding, it often comes with its share of stress, anxiety, and fatigue. I think of respite as "one step backward, two steps forward," allowing us to keep making steady progress toward our goals. Here are a few key reasons why respite is not just a luxury but a necessity:

1. **Preventing Burnout:** Constantly being "on duty" can lead to caregiver burnout, a state of emotional, physical, and mental exhaustion. Burnout can manifest as feelings of resentment, frustration, and even depression. Taking breaks allows fathers to step away from the pressures of caregiving, helping to prevent burnout and maintain emotional health.

2. **Improving Relationships:** When caregivers are constantly stressed, their relationships can suffer. Taking time for oneself allows fathers to return to their families rejuvenated, emotionally available, and better equipped to engage with their partners and children. Respite can also provide an opportunity for couples to reconnect, strengthening their partnership amid the challenges of parenting.

3. **Enhancing Effectiveness:** Research shows that rested and renewed individuals are more effective in their roles. When fathers take breaks, they can return to their responsibilities with a clearer mind, better focus, and more energy. This renewed approach not only benefits the individual but ultimately enhances the family dynamic.

4. **Promoting Self-Care:** Respite is a critical component of self-care. It provides fathers the chance to engage in activities that nurture their interests, hobbies, and passions—elements that may have taken a back seat during the caregiving journey. Prioritizing respite is a way of honoring one's own needs, leading to a more balanced life.

Overcoming Guilt: Embracing the Need for Breaks

One of the most significant barriers a father faces when considering respite is guilt. The idea of taking time away from caregiving can feel selfish, especially when you believe your child needs your presence. However, it's essential to shift this mindset and recognize that prioritizing your own well-being ultimately benefits the entire family.

Reframing Guilt into Empowerment

1. **Recognize the Value of Self-Care:** Understanding that your well-being is crucial for your ability to care for your child is the first step in overcoming guilt. When you prioritize self-care, you are not only recharging your own batteries but also setting a positive example for your children about the importance of personal well-being.
2. **Challenge Negative Thoughts:** Guilt often stems from internalized beliefs about parenting and masculinity. Challenge the notion that taking breaks makes you a less dedicated father. Instead, remind yourself that caring for your own needs enables you to be a better, more engaged parent.
3. **Communicate Openly:** Discuss your need for breaks with your partner and family members. Open communication can help foster a supportive environment where everyone understands the importance of respite. Engaging in this dialogue can also promote teamwork, where both parents feel empowered to take time for self-care.
4. **Prioritize Quality over Quantity:** Respite doesn't always have to mean long periods away from home. Sometimes, it can be as simple as taking an hour each week to engage in an activity you love. Focus on the quality of your time away, rather than the quantity.

Practical Strategies for Finding Respite

Finding time for respite given the demands of parenting can be challenging, but with some creativity and planning, it is achievable. We all get the same 24 hours a day or 168 hours per week. How we invest or spend our time is a personal choice. Here are some practical strategies for integrating breaks into your life:

1. Schedule Regular Breaks

Treat your breaks as appointments that cannot be missed. By intentionally scheduling regular respite time into your calendar, you create a commitment to your self-care.

- **Daily Micro-Breaks:** Even just ten to fifteen minutes each day can make a difference. Use this time for deep breathing exercises, a short walk, or simply enjoying a cup of coffee in silence. For dads who commute to and from work, be intentional about using these nuggets of time as wisely as possible. Would listening to a book on Audible or your favorite podcasts provide some enjoyment?
- **Weekly Mini-Breaks:** Set aside a few hours each week to engage in an activity that brings you joy, such as fishing, golfing, or visiting friends. There is a direct correlation to the way we budget our time and financial resources and the activities we pursue. Many of the SFN Mastermind Group dads think of the weekly meetings as a critical part of their weekly respite plan. Spending time in a safe and encouraging environment with like-minded dads will have a dramatic impact on your well-being. You can learn more about the SFN Mastermind Groups in Chapter 11.
- **Monthly Meetups:** Some dads prefer to meet monthly since there is a more modest time commitment. While you're unlikely to get to know others as deeply, getting together with like-minded dads monthly might be a good way to connect. Traditionally these groups have met at a restaurant or a bar and are a bit more social. One good example of a successful monthly meetup group is Dads Appreciating Down Syndrome (DADS) started in Indianapolis, Indiana, with chapters in more than forty locations around the US.

Tom Delaney of Downers Grove, Illinois, a local leader of DADS-Chicago, and **Lyle Liechty**, one of the original cofounders of DADS in Indianapolis, Indiana, have impacted hundreds of dads who have children with Down syndrome.

> *One of the most important decisions I made was getting involved with the DADS group that we have, because it put me into a network of fathers who understand and can relate to what I'm going through. Some of the greatest guys in the world. I mean, they're so courageous and they're strong and their perspective is amazing.*
>
> *And just off-the-charts good guys, their ability to maintain their sense of humor in the face of some pretty challenging circumstances. I'm inspired by them. I'm inspired by the guys in the group every day and it pays me back. I feel like it's a good thing that I'm involved in.*
>
> —Tom Delaney, *Dad To Dad Podcast*, episode #44

> *DADS actually stands for Dads Appreciating Down Syndrome.*
>
> *So we formed a group, there were seven or eight of us that formed DADS. It was great because we all had newborns or young, very young children. And so that started about twenty-two years ago and we'd meet on the second Tuesday of the month at a restaurant and we would talk and share, and then it evolved to having speakers come in that would be applicable to different things you know, physical therapy companies or pediatricians or a financial planner. You know, we've had every type of profession that we can think of that would be helpful to speak to our DADS group. And we continue that, probably nine or ten months of the year we have a speaker. The other two or three we just have dads sharing stories, which is valuable because it helps connect or maybe answer questions that you have instead of trying to navigate the world by yourself.*
>
> —Lyle Liechty, *Dad To Dad Podcast*, episode #139

2. Utilize Respite Care Services

Many communities offer respite care services tailored for families with special needs. These programs can provide temporary relief for caregivers, allowing fathers (and mothers) to take a break while ensuring their child is in safe, caring hands.

- **In-Home Respite:** Consider hiring a caregiver to provide support at home. This can allow you to run errands, take a nap, or enjoy a personal hobby while knowing your child is well cared for.
- **Day Programs:** Some organizations offer day programs for children or adults with special needs. Enrolling your child in one of these programs can provide you with several hours of respite.
- **Overnight and Short-Term Respite Care:** Finding a program for medically fragile children in a home-like setting with trained staff and equipment is very difficult. Children's Respite Homes of America is a US-based network committed to developing overnight respite homes for medically complex children. One example is **A Rosie Place for Children** in South Bend, Indiana, a nonprofit, licensed specialty hospital and respite facility that serves children who are medically fragile, including those dependent on ventilators, feeding tubes, or other intensive medical supports. The facility offers stays of three to ten nights, free of charge to Indiana families, during which the child receives high-level nursing and medically complex care in a "home-away-from-home" environment, while caregivers get much-needed relief.

A Rosie Place for Children founder **Tieal Bishop** of Walkerton, Indiana, is a pioneer and visionary leader.

> *A Rosie Place for Children is just this extraordinary, magical place. We don't like to call it a home. We don't like to call it a facility. It's actually licensed as a hospital because we wanted the highest level of care. But we try not to function like that on the outside because we don't want it to seem so clinical or sterile.*
>
> —Tieal Bishop, *Dad To Dad Podcast*, episode #356

3. Engage Family and Friends

Don't hesitate to lean on your support network. Family and friends can be invaluable resources for respite care. While not everyone is trustworthy or has prior experience, who within your family or friend group can you approach?

- **Family Support:** Reach out to relatives who may be willing to spend time with your child. Grandparents, aunts, and uncles often

enjoy being involved in their lives and can provide temporary relief for you.
- **Friend Exchanges:** If you have friends in similar situations, consider arranging reciprocal care. Offer to care for their children while they take a break, and in return, they can do the same for you.

4. Explore Community Resources

Many communities have organizations that offer resources, support, and programs for families with special needs. Research local options to find respite programs or support groups that can help provide relief.
- **Support Groups:** Connecting with local support groups for fathers can be an excellent way to share experiences, gain insight, and explore respite options together.
- **Community Centers:** Many community centers offer recreational programs specifically designed for children with special needs. Participating in these programs can offer opportunities for both children and parents to enjoy some well-deserved breaks.

Activities for Personal Renewal

Taking time for yourself is essential, but it's equally important to engage in activities that promote personal renewal. Here are some ideas for activities that can help you recharge:

1. Physical Activity

Exercise is not just a way to stay physically healthy; it also has a significant impact on mental and emotional well-being. Find an activity that you enjoy and make it part of your routine.
- **Group Classes:** Joining a local gym or fitness class can provide both physical activity and social connection. Look for classes that fit your interests, such as cycling, yoga, or martial arts.
- **Working with Your Hands:** Many guys find working on their cars, tinkering in a home workshop, or gardening to be a healthy way to gain some "me time."
- **Outdoor Activities:** Enjoying nature can be a great way to relax and recharge. Outdoor activities such as hiking, biking, or simply taking a walk in the park can help clear your mind.

2. Creative Pursuits

Engaging in creative activities allows you to express yourself and tap into your passions. Creativity can be a powerful outlet for stress relief.

- **Art and Craft Projects:** Whether you enjoy painting, drawing, or crafting, engaging in artistic pursuits can be therapeutic. Don't worry about the end result—just focus on the process and let your creativity flow.
- **Writing or Journaling:** Writing can be an effective way to process your thoughts and emotions. Consider starting a journal where you can reflect on your experiences, express gratitude, or simply write freely about your day. Consider **Andy McCall** in Greenville, Tennessee, whose daughter, Penelope, was born with special needs and then got cancer. Penelope died before her second birthday. Andy kept a blog, which he turned into a book entitled *Pigtails & Steel*. While not everyone's journals or blogs will morph into a book, the exercise of writing or journaling can be very therapeutic.

Ellen and I talked about it, and she goes, you should share it and just share it to Facebook. Maybe somebody will read it. And maybe, you know, somebody will know what we're going through. And it sort of went like wildfire from there.

People were reading my thoughts. And I wasn't really good at first, communicating how I felt. You know, a lot of people didn't know how to talk to me about things or even what I was thinking about this whole situation. I put it out there and just put my thoughts at the time. And it not only helped me. It helped my family. It helped Ellen. It helped some other people going through this. And like I said, I just kept going until about a year after Penelope died.

—**Andy McCall**, *Dad To Dad Podcast*, **episode #144**

3. Social Connections

Building and maintaining social connections is crucial for emotional well-being. Making time to connect with friends can provide valuable support and a much-needed break. Research by the Survey Center on American Life reveals the typical guy has only five friends, three close friends and two best friends. Maintaining relationships with guys from high school or college, outside of work, or even with guys in the neighborhood means being more intentional.

- **Regular Meetups:** Schedule regular outings with other couples or friends, whether it's for coffee, dinner, or a fun activity. Having these social engagements can offer a refreshing change of pace. Just having a date on the calendar that you're looking forward to provides a psychological benefit.

Don Raineri of Downers Grove, Illinois, helped start Dads of Steele, a support group for dads who lost a child.

> *He just had this vision of creating this organization that would bring dads together to motivate them, to encourage them, and to inspire each other.*
>
> *So it's become a, you know, a place where dads can come together. They can share their successes. They can also share their struggles and they can do that in a safe place basically. The whole vision is that we want dads to become the best version of themselves that they can be for their families.*
>
> —**Don Raineri,** *Dad To Dad Podcast,* **episode #138**

- **Supportive Conversations:** Sometimes, simply talking with someone who understands your journey can be incredibly rejuvenating. Whether it's a close friend or a fellow father in a similar situation, be intentional and make time for meaningful conversations.

Encouraging a Culture of Respite in Your Family

As fathers, we play a critical role in shaping the dynamics of our families. By modeling the importance of respite, we can encourage our partners and children to recognize the value of self-care as well. Here's how to cultivate a family culture that embraces breaks and renewal:

1. **Normalize the Need for Breaks:** Openly discuss the importance of taking breaks with your family. Emphasize that everyone has needs and that prioritizing self-care is a healthy choice for everyone involved.
2. **Create Family Respite Plans:** Involve your family in creating a respite plan. Encourage open discussions about when and how

each family member can take time for themselves. Consider scheduling regular family outings or individual time for each member.
3. **Share the Load:** Encourage your partner and children to share responsibilities. By distributing tasks among family members, everyone can have the opportunity for respite, creating a more balanced environment.
4. **Celebrate Individual Time:** Acknowledge and celebrate the moments when family members take time for themselves. Whether it's a child pursuing a hobby or your partner engaging in a self-care routine, recognize these efforts as valuable contributions to family well-being.

Conclusion: Embracing Respite for a Stronger Family

In the demanding journey of raising a child with special needs, prioritizing respite is not just an act of self-care; it is an essential component of a healthy family dynamic. By embracing breaks without guilt and recognizing their importance, fathers can cultivate resilience, emotional well-being, and stronger relationships with their families.

Respite allows fathers to return to their roles with renewed energy and perspective, enabling them to face challenges with greater strength. As you navigate this journey, remember that taking care of yourself is not selfish; it's an investment in your family's future. By nurturing your own well-being, you're creating a supportive, balanced environment where both you and your child can thrive.

So, give yourself permission to take a break. Embrace the power of respite and remember that your own renewal is key to being the father your child needs.

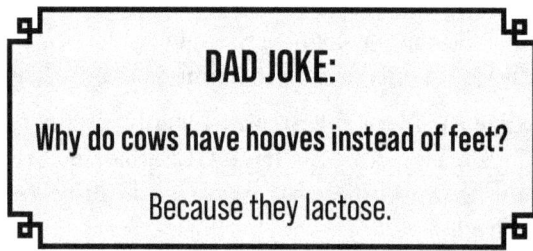

- 8 -
Faith and Fatherhood: Spirituality as a Guide on the Special Needs Journey

FAITH-FILLED STEP

Through trials deep, through nights so long,
My love stays fierce, my heart stays strong.
Though paths are rough, though storms may rise,
I see the world through hopeful eyes.

With steady hands, I lift, I guide,
Faith walks with me, right by my side.

Disclaimer: Spirituality can be a meaningful source of comfort, strength, and perspective, but it isn't the right path for everyone. Each person's beliefs, experiences, and values shape what resonates with them. Individuals should explore only what feels authentic and supportive to their own journey. If you're a dyed-in-the-wool atheist, it's okay to skip this chapter. If you're unsure or curious to learn more about the role of spirituality, I hope you find this chapter of value.

The journey of parenting a child with special needs often leads fathers down a path of profound reflection, introspection, and transformation. As they navigate the complexities of advocacy, education, and caregiving, many fathers find themselves grappling with existential questions about purpose, meaning, and the essence of life itself. For some, spirituality and faith emerge as a source of strength, guidance, and solace amid the challenges. This chapter explores the intersection of faith and fatherhood, examining how spirituality can serve as a compass on the journey of raising a child with special needs.

The Role of Faith in Parenting

Faith can take many forms and varies significantly among individuals. For some, it is rooted in organized religion; for others, it manifests in personal beliefs, spiritual practices, or a connection to something greater than oneself. Regardless of its form, faith can provide fathers with a framework for understanding their experiences and navigating the challenges they face.

Let's address the eight-hundred-pound gorilla in the room. Many individuals experience a crisis of faith. Getting a diagnosis of a disability or serious medical condition for a child is, in some cases, the biggest challenge a parent will experience. The most common refrain is "How could God let this happen to my child or our family?" This is normal and experienced by a large percentage of parents. It's not a punishment for something you did or didn't do; it's just life.

Take **Greg Hubert** of Torrence, California, who has three boys with autism. He and his wife both went through a crisis of faith. In his case, it led to a career shift from the corporate world to serving the disability community, initially with Joni and Friends, the global Christian disability ministry helping people with disabilities and their families, and now with the Brookwood Community, a Christian residential and vocational community for those with disabilities, in Brookside, Texas.

> *And then sure enough, little Tate was diagnosed with autism in a similar way. So, we had the trifecta of autism in our family. All three of the boys diagnosed with autism spectrum disorder.*
>
> —Greg Hubert, ***Dad To Dad Podcast***, episode #172

Finding Meaning in Difficult Circumstances

When a child is born with special needs, it can be challenging to comprehend the complexities and difficulties that come with the diagnosis. Many fathers may question why their child has these challenges and what it means for their family. This goes beyond being in denial. Here are some catchphrases to alert yourself to the situation, which I often say: "Let's not pre-worry our worries," "We'll cross that bridge when we get there," and "Some kids just take longer to reach a milestone."

Faith can help answer these questions and offer a deeper understanding of these circumstances.

- **Embracing the Unknown:** Faith encourages acceptance of uncertainty. While it may not provide concrete answers to why certain challenges arise, it fosters a sense of peace in knowing that life is

filled with mysteries. This acceptance can help fathers find strength during their struggles.
- **Seeking Purpose:** Many fathers find that their experiences lead them to seek greater meaning and purpose in life. Spiritual beliefs can provide a framework for understanding suffering and hardship, transforming challenges into opportunities for growth and learning.

Spiritual Practices for Fathers

Engaging in spiritual practices can be a powerful way to connect with one's faith and find solace during challenging times. Here are some spiritual practices that fathers can incorporate into their lives to support their journey:

1. Prayer and Meditation

For many, prayer is a vital aspect of spiritual life. It provides a direct line of communication with the divine and allows for reflection, gratitude, and the expression of hopes and fears. Similarly, meditation can help fathers cultivate mindfulness and present-moment awareness.

- **Creating a Routine:** Setting aside specific times for prayer or meditation can provide a grounding ritual in daily life. Whether taking a few minutes in the morning, during lunch breaks, or before bed, these moments of reflection can offer a respite from the challenges of caregiving.
- **Finding Community:** Engaging in group prayer or meditation can foster a sense of community and support. Many spiritual organizations offer group gatherings where individuals can share their experiences and find collective strength.

2. Reading Sacred Texts

Many fathers find comfort and guidance in the teachings of sacred texts, whether they come from religious scripture or philosophical writings. These texts often offer profound insights into the nature of love, compassion, and resilience.

- **Daily Reflection:** Set aside time to read and reflect on passages that resonate with your experiences. Journaling your thoughts can help you process and internalize the messages you encounter. When I converted to Christianity in 2011, one of the gifts I received from Charlie Bale, a dear friend and client, was a copy of *Jesus Calling* by Sarah Young. I have literally read a page a day, before bed, every year for the past fifteen years. Another gift was the suggestion about keeping a gratitude journal. Research studies support that journaling and a nightly reflection ritual help calm the mind by reducing stress, organizing thoughts, and signaling the body that it's time to unwind. These practices strengthen emotional resilience by promoting reflection, gratitude, and healthier processing of daily experiences. Over time, they improve sleep quality, boost mental clarity, and contribute to greater overall well-being. The routine of journaling and reflecting on a scripture passage before falling asleep has been a cornerstone of my daily routine.

- **Exploring Different Perspectives:** Delving into various spiritual or philosophical texts can provide new insights and perspectives. Exploring the writings of different faith traditions can enrich your understanding and expand your spiritual toolkit. My friend **Eboo Patel**, founder and president of Interfaith America, has been a great source of knowledge and insight as it relates to all things interfaith. I can highly recommend two of his books: *Act of Faith* and *Sacred Ground*.

3. Nature as a Spiritual Guide

Nature can serve as a profound source of inspiration and connection to spirituality. Spending time outdoors can help fathers reflect on their experiences and connect with the world around them.

- **Mindful Walks**: Take regular walks in nature, allowing yourself to be present in the moment. Observe the beauty of your surroundings, and let the sights, sounds, and scents ground you in the present.
- **Creating Rituals:** Consider establishing rituals that connect you with nature. This could involve gardening, hiking, or simply sitting in a park. Allow these moments to be a form of worship and appreciation for the world around you.
- **For Those Who Are More Athletic:** Consider cycling, running, or swimming as three examples of combining an athletic endeavor and being outdoors. Or consider combining all three and pursue triathlons. I did my first Olympic distance triathlon, 1.5-kilometer swim, a 40-kilometer bike ride, and a 10-kilometer run, when I

was 28. My time was pathetically slow, and at the time I checked triathlon off my "To-Do List." It wasn't until I was 36 when the triathlon bug really bit me, and I started doing one or two triathlons a year: mostly Olympic distance, then occasionally half Ironman events, before doing my first Ironman distance triathlon, Ironman Wisconsin, at age 49. When I turned 60, I decided to see if I still had some gas left in the tank and completed Ironman Florida. Taking a page out of George H. W. Bush's playbook (who went skydiving with the US Army Golden Knights at 50, 60, 70, and 80), my ambition is to do another Ironman at 70 and, God willing, again at 80. If I have to explain why, you wouldn't understand.

The Importance of Community and Support

Faith often thrives in community. For fathers of children with special needs, connecting with others who share similar experiences can provide valuable support, encouragement, and understanding.

1. Joining Support Groups

Many communities offer faith-based support groups for families with special needs. These groups can serve as a safe space for fathers to share their struggles, fears, and triumphs.

- **Finding Connection:** Joining a group of like-minded dads can help fathers feel less isolated and more understood. Hearing the stories of others can foster a sense of belonging and solidarity.
- **Learning from Others:** Groups of like-minded dads often provide valuable insights and practical tips for navigating the challenges of parenting a child with special needs. The shared wisdom of others can be a powerful resource.

2. Engaging in Faith Communities

Faith communities, whether churches, synagogues, or spiritual centers, can provide a supportive network for fathers. Many religious organizations offer programs specifically designed to assist families with special needs.

- **Inclusive Programs:** Seek out faith communities that prioritize inclusivity and support for families with special needs. These organizations often offer programs, resources, and community outreach that can be invaluable.

Skip Gianopulos, one of my longtime friends and neighbors, has been involved with the Special Friends program at Willow Creek Community Church in South Barrington, Illinois. All four of his girls, the two with Down syndrome and their typical sisters, have been involved in an annual stage production of musicals including *The Wizard of Oz*, *Aladdin Jr.*, and *Frozen Jr.*

> *There are days when our special needs kids are a whole lot easier than our typical kids.*
>
> *Particularly with Down syndrome, there's no predisposition to having a second child with Down syndrome once you have your first. So literally, it's like lightning striking twice. In fact, I thought a little bit about buying lottery tickets after that.*
>
> —Skip Gianopulos, *Dad To Dad Podcast*, episode #4

- **Volunteer Opportunities:** Engaging in volunteer work within your faith community can provide a sense of purpose and fulfillment. Helping others can foster gratitude and appreciation for the blessings in your life. I have two favorite organizations. The first is **Habitat for Humanity**, which I was first involved with in 1990 and virtually every year since. The second is **Joni and Friends**, one of the oldest and largest global Christian disability ministries. Joni and Friends offers family retreats, which are worthy of your consideration, and I love their **Wheels for the World (WFTW)** program that collects, refurbishes, and distributes wheelchairs to forty destinations in twenty-five countries. My wife and I traveled to Bayamo, Cuba, with WFTW in April 2024 and distributed more than two hundred wheelchairs. Here are some pearls of wisdom from my Joni and Friends SFN Mentor Fathers: **Steve Bundy, Jon Ebersole, John Fela,** and **Greg Hubert.**

> *In the early years of fatherhood with a special needs son, I was looking for guidance. I was looking for a path. I really didn't find anyone in my journey who had gone before me—someone who had been on a similar path—to come alongside me, mentor me, and assure me that not all is lost....*
>
> *I wish somebody had been there for me. And if I can be that mentor to another young father—man, I'm there. I look forward to doing that.*
>
> —**Steve Bundy,** *Dad To Dad Podcast,* **episode #34**

> *All five of us in my family understand that we would not be who we are today were it not for disability. None of us like that Amanda and Jessica have disabilities, and yet that's the reality.*
>
> *As Joni Eareckson Tada says, sometimes disability sandblasts our souls—it jackhammers away pride and fear. And I would not be who I am today were it not for disability.*
>
> —**Jon Ebersole,** *Dad To Dad Podcast,* **episode #46**

> *Being in the waiting room they gave us, I was really just praying to God:* **Whatever you need to take from me to heal him, I'm willing to give you. Whatever that is—you can have it all, if it means my son will be healed.**
>
> *In that moment, it took me back to when we struggled the most as a family. I was willing to give everything up.* **Please—just heal my child.**
>
> —**John Fela,** *Dad To Dad Podcast,* **episode #65**

> *The behaviors—the things our boys did when they couldn't talk—those meltdowns. When they knew Mommy and Daddy were spending time together and that we were good, you saw those behaviors drastically minimized.*
>
> *They didn't completely go away, but you could sense it, David. When we were good with each other, the boys were good.*
>
> —**Greg Hubert,** *Dad To Dad Podcast,* **episode #144**

Navigating Spiritual Challenges

While faith can be a source of strength, it's essential to acknowledge that spiritual challenges may arise on the journey. Fathers may experience feelings of anger, doubt, or frustration, particularly during difficult times. Navigating these challenges is a normal part of the spiritual journey.

1. Addressing Doubts and Questions

Have you experienced a "crisis of faith?" It's natural for fathers to question their faith or beliefs, especially when faced with overwhelming circumstances. Instead of suppressing these feelings, it's essential to acknowledge and explore them.

- **Open Conversations:** Discuss your doubts and questions with trusted friends, mentors, or spiritual leaders. Engaging in honest conversations can help you process your feelings and find clarity.
- **Reflective Journaling:** Consider journaling about your spiritual doubts and questions. Writing can be a powerful way to explore your thoughts and feelings, allowing you to gain deeper insights.

2. Embracing Vulnerability

Being vulnerable is a fundamental aspect of the spiritual journey. Historically, most men have thought that being vulnerable is a weakness. More enlightened men understand embracing vulnerability is a strength. It allows fathers to connect with their true selves and with others authentically.

- **Sharing Experiences:** Sharing your experiences, struggles, and triumphs with trusted individuals can create deeper connections and foster a sense of community. Vulnerability can also inspire others to be more open about their journeys.

Paul Peterangelo of Tonawanda, New York, leads a virtual Bible study group of special needs dads from across the US and beyond.

> *I can tell you that Amanda has made every single person in our family—bar none—better human beings. Because in her, we really see what God wants us all to do, which is to love one another unconditionally.*
>
> *Regardless of developmental status. Regardless of color. Regardless of race. It doesn't matter to her. And consequently, it's never mattered to any of my kids either.*
>
> —**Paul Peterangelo**, *Dad To Dad Podcast*, **episode #246**

- **Seeking Support:** Don't hesitate to seek support from spiritual leaders or counselors who specialize in faith-related issues. They can provide guidance and help you navigate spiritual challenges with compassion.

Celebrating Spiritual Milestones

Just as milestones in a child's development are worth celebrating, so, too, are the spiritual milestones fathers achieve along the way. Recognizing and honoring these moments can deepen the connection to one's faith.

1. Acknowledging Growth

Take time to reflect on your spiritual growth throughout the journey of fatherhood. Acknowledge how your experiences have shaped your beliefs and values.

- **Personal Rituals:** Consider creating personal rituals that celebrate your spiritual milestones. This could involve lighting a candle, writing a letter to your future self, or participating in a ceremony that honors your growth.
- **Gratitude Practices:** Incorporate gratitude practices into your daily routine. Regularly reflecting on what you are thankful for can deepen your connection to spirituality and enhance your overall well-being. As mentioned previously, I have been journaling daily with things I'm thankful for during the past fifteen years.

2. Engaging in Service

Service to others can be a profound expression of faith and spirituality. Many fathers find that giving back to their communities helps them feel more connected to their purpose.

- **Volunteer Work:** Explore volunteer opportunities that resonate with your values and passions. Helping others can provide a sense of fulfillment and deepen your spiritual journey. Quite a few SFN Mentor Fathers have created nonprofit organizations and pour dozens of hours a month into them volunteering. The comment I hear most often is how "therapeutic" volunteering is. I can personally vouch for that, having founded and led two fatherhood nonprofit organizations. Take the *SFN Dad To Dad Podcast* for example. I typically invest five to ten hours preparing for each episode. That's two hundred fifty to five hundred hours a year making sure I'm well prepared to record a brief conversation with each guest. Getting your mind off your own situation and concentrating on giving back is a sure way to develop mental fitness.
- **Family Involvement:** Encourage your children to participate in service activities as well. Engaging in acts of kindness as a family can strengthen your bond and cultivate a spirit of compassion. One of the most rewarding projects I helped create and lead for the better part of a decade was the Youth Advisory Council of the **Barrington Area Community Foundation** in Barrington, Illinois. The group consisted of twenty high school students, five per grade. The purpose was to help educate them about philanthropy. We held monthly meetings, read and discussed books, and organized an annual food drive, as well as holding a fundraiser. The highlight of the year was organizing an annual field trip and taking the students into Chicago where we would visit foundations, meeting nonprofit leaders and usually attending a luncheon with a featured speaker. My younger three kids were involved with the group over the course of about seven years. While this was a lot of work, I found it very rewarding to provide a small group of future leaders with some insights about philanthropy, a world that most adults don't ever get a chance to experience.

The Impact of Spirituality on Family Dynamics

Spirituality can significantly influence family dynamics and create a supportive environment for all family members. Fathers who embrace their spirituality often model resilience, compassion, and gratitude for their children. After retiring, **Rick Bolle** of Naperville, Illinois, was called to create Front Porch Church, an inclusive weekly worship community intentionally designed to welcome individuals of all abilities and their families, emphasizing that everyone is seen, valued, and loved in their journey toward God.

> *There might be shouting or dancing in the aisles, but at Front Porch Church, there are no distractions—only interactions within our community.*
>
> *That really lays the groundwork for understanding that it's not about "You have to sit here and be quiet." We'll have a young boy come up and play with Lydia, our worship director, on stage. He'll bring his guitar. And we don't say no.*
>
> *We want to include everybody. We just don't say no.*
>
> —Rick Bolle, *Dad To Dad Podcast*, episode #381

1. Instilling Values

By embracing spirituality, fathers can instill core values in their children that promote empathy, understanding, and acceptance.

- **Modeling Behavior:** Demonstrating compassion, kindness, and gratitude in everyday life can help children develop similar values. Children learn by example, and fathers who prioritize their spirituality can influence their children's outlook on life.
- **Family Discussions:** Encourage open discussions about spirituality and values within the family. Engaging in conversations about beliefs, morals, and ethics can create a safe space for children to explore their own spirituality.

2. Building Resilience

Fathers who draw on their spirituality often develop greater resilience in the face of challenges. This resilience can be a powerful tool for the entire family.

- **Emotional Support:** Providing emotional support and understanding helps children navigate their own challenges. Fathers who embody resilience can inspire their children to cultivate strength in difficult times.
- **Problem-Solving Skills:** Teaching children how to approach challenges with a spiritual perspective can equip them with

valuable problem-solving skills. Encourage them to seek guidance, reflect, and find meaning in their experiences.

Conclusion: The Journey of Faith and Fatherhood

Navigating the journey of raising a child with special needs can be both rewarding and challenging. Throughout this journey, spirituality can serve as a guiding force, providing fathers with strength, purpose, and a sense of belonging. By engaging in spiritual practices, seeking support, and addressing challenges, fathers can deepen their connection to their faith and to their families.

Ultimately, embracing faith as a guiding principle can empower fathers to approach their role with resilience, compassion, and love. As they navigate the complexities of raising a child with special needs, fathers can find solace and inspiration in their spirituality, transforming challenges into opportunities for growth.

As you embark on your journey, remember that faith and fatherhood are intertwined. Let spirituality be your guide, helping you navigate the ups and downs of life with grace, purpose, and unwavering love.

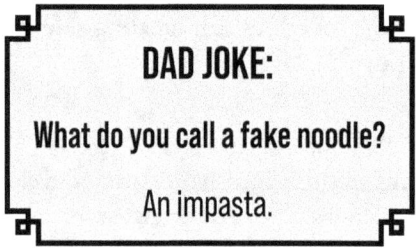

- 9 -
Siblings Matter: Balancing Attention and Love Across the Entire Family

FATHERING ALL MY CHILDREN

Between the needs, the love, the care,
I split my time, though never fair.
One child's world spins fast, so bright,
The other's calls fade into night.

Yet in their eyes, I see they know,
Love still finds its way to show.
A hand, a hug, a whispered cheer—
I am their father, always near.

In the intricate tapestry of family life, each member plays a vital role, and the presence of siblings adds a unique dimension to the dynamics of love, support, and growth. When a child with special needs enters the picture, the balance of attention and love within the family can shift dramatically. While the needs of the child with special abilities may require a considerable amount of focus and care, it is crucial not to overlook the emotional and developmental needs of siblings. This chapter will explore the significance of siblings in the family, the challenges they may face, and strategies for ensuring that all children feel valued, heard, and loved.

The Unique Role of Siblings

Siblings share a bond that is unlike any other relationship in life. They often serve as confidants, playmates, and, in many cases, lifelong friends. In families with children who have special needs, siblings can have unique experiences and perspectives that contribute to their personal development.

Here are a couple poignant passages from siblings who did interviews for the *SFN Dad To Dad Podcast*:

Bill Danko is a retired professor at University at Albany, State University of New York (SUNY Albany) and *New York Times* best-selling author. Sadly, Bill's dad, Milton, a WWII veteran, died at 38 from multiple sclerosis, and his younger brother, Tony, was diagnosed at 21 with MS. After Bill's mom passed away, Bill became the sole caregiver to Tony, who died in 2015 at age 68. Bill shares some poignant insights about the importance of sibling relationships.

> *That's a joy. And likewise, when you have the opportunity—like I had with my brother—you see how much attitude matters. He had a good attitude. He was a faithful man. Spirituality and religion were important to him.*
>
> *I don't think he could have survived as long as he did without that faith. I truly believe that. Was he ever upset or despondent? Yes. But you get through it. He had a good attitude.*
>
> —**Bill Danko**, *Dad To Dad Podcast*, episode #125

Rob Johnson is a seven-time Emmy Award–winning broadcast journalist and an outspoken advocate for those with disabilities. His younger brother, Edward, has Down syndrome. Informed by his close relationship with Edward, Rob has become a strong advocate for families touched by Down syndrome and other disabilities.

> *You know, he agrees with everything, so you can't ask him yes-or-no questions.*
>
> *"Edward, everything going okay?"*
>
> *"Yeah."*
>
> *"Edward, is the sky green?"*
>
> *"Yeah."*
>
> *He'll agree with you on everything, so you really can't ask yes-or-no questions. But he has such a wonderful soul. Learning about people with disabilities—through my brother, and then meeting other kids back then who are now young and older adults—that's really where it all started for me.*
>
> —**Rob Johnson**, *Dad To Dad Podcast*, episode #133

1. Companionship and Emotional Support

Siblings often provide one another with companionship and a sense of belonging. For a child with special needs, having a sibling can enhance their social skills and emotional well-being.

- **Mutual Understanding:** Siblings can often relate to each other's experiences, leading to a strong bond of understanding. A sibling's ability to empathize with their brother or sister's challenges fosters a deeper connection.
- **Emotional Outlet:** Siblings often act as emotional outlets for each other. When a child with special needs is facing challenges, their sibling may offer support or a listening ear, which can be invaluable for emotional processing.

2. Learning Opportunities

Siblings can be powerful teachers, offering insights and skills that promote growth and understanding.

- **Social Skills Development:** Interacting with a sibling who has special needs can enhance social skills, including communication, patience, and empathy. Siblings learn to navigate differences and develop adaptability as they engage in diverse interactions.
- **Understanding Differences:** Growing up with a sibling who has special needs allows children to learn about diversity and acceptance from an early age. This experience can foster open-mindedness and compassion, shaping their attitudes toward others in society.

Challenges Faced by Siblings

While the bond between siblings can be incredibly rewarding, it can also present challenges, particularly when one child has special needs. These challenges may affect their emotional, social, and developmental well-being.

1. Feelings of Neglect

Siblings of children with special needs may feel overlooked or neglected due to the heightened attention that the child with special needs often receives. This can lead to feelings of resentment or inadequacy.

- **Seeking Attention:** Siblings may act out or engage in attention-seeking behaviors to compete for parental focus. They may feel

that their accomplishments and needs are less important, leading to frustration and sadness.
- **Emotional Strain:** The emotional toll of feeling secondary can result in anxiety, depression, or behavioral issues in siblings. It is vital to recognize and address these feelings to foster a supportive family environment.

2. Caregiver Role

In some families, siblings may inadvertently take on a caregiving role, leading to increased pressure and responsibility at a young age.

- **Mature Responsibilities:** Older siblings may feel the need to step in and help care for their sibling with special needs, taking on tasks that are often beyond their emotional capacity. This can hinder their own childhood experiences and personal development.
- **Burden of Responsibility:** The sense of responsibility for their sibling's well-being can lead to stress and anxiety, making it difficult for siblings to focus on their own needs and aspirations.

3. Trauma

Many siblings who have a brother or sister with a disability may grow up watching their sibling self-injure, or they may have been the victims of their sibling's aggression, which can be very difficult. Also, siblings of brothers or sisters with complex medical issues may see their brother or sister experience extreme medical emergencies on a routine basis, which can also be distressing.

- **Possible Post-Traumatic Stress Disorder:** These experiences may result in the sibling having flashbacks of distressing events, high levels of anxiety, negative thoughts and beliefs, hypervigilance, nightmares, or other symptoms that may disrupt their lives.
- **Ambivalence Toward the Sibling:** Most brothers and sisters love their sibling with special needs, but for those who exhibit self-injury or aggression, the typical sibling may also fear their brother or sister, which can create internal turmoil. They may also experience guilt if they have had to fight back to defend themselves or another sibling or parent.
- **Fear of Losing the Sibling:** For those who have a brother or sister with severe medical complications, they may live with an underlying fear that the sibling could be gone at any time.

Balancing Attention and Love

To ensure that all children in the family feel valued and supported, it is important to be intentional about establishing a balance of attention and love. Here are some strategies to foster an inclusive family environment that nurtures the needs of all children.

1. One-on-One Time

Carving out dedicated time for each child can strengthen bonds and create a sense of security.

- **Individual Activities:** Engage in activities that allow for one-on-one interactions with each child. Whether it's going for ice cream, playing a game, or simply talking, these moments can help children feel prioritized and appreciated.
- **Scheduled Family Meetings:** Consider setting up regular family meetings where each child can express their thoughts and feelings. This platform fosters open communication and ensures everyone's voice is heard.
- **Take and Frame Photos:** Family memories are largely burnished by photographic images. While memories may fade or get distorted, photos have a way of timestamping our experiences. Whether you frame them or create Shutterfly photo albums, doing so will help enhance the collective legacy of time spent with each of your family members.

2. Open Communication

Fostering open and honest communication within the family is essential for addressing the needs and emotions of each child.

- **Encouraging Expression:** Create an environment where siblings feel comfortable expressing their thoughts and emotions. Encourage them to share their feelings about their sibling's needs and the family dynamics. Not doing so risks these feelings manifesting in ways that have the potential to undermine healthy relationships.
- **Active Listening:** Practice active listening when siblings share their concerns or experiences. Acknowledging their feelings can validate their experiences and reinforce their importance in the family. As an example: "What I heard you say..."

3. Inclusion in Caregiving

Involving siblings in the caregiving process can foster a sense of unity and understanding.

- **Collaborative Activities:** Include siblings in activities that support their sibling with special needs, such as homework, playtime, or therapy sessions, if the sibling is willing to help. This can promote teamwork and understanding among siblings.
- **Highlighting Strengths:** Acknowledge and celebrate the strengths that siblings bring to the caregiving process. Highlighting their contributions fosters a sense of pride and belonging.

Celebrating Differences and Abilities

One of the most important aspects of balancing attention and love across the family is embracing the unique strengths and abilities of each child.

1. Celebrating Individual Achievements

Recognizing and celebrating each child's achievements, regardless of their abilities, can foster a sense of pride and accomplishment.

- **Personalized Recognition:** Create personalized recognition for each child's achievements, big or small. Whether you offer awards, hold family celebrations, or simply provide verbal affirmations, acknowledging their efforts can boost self-esteem.
- **Family Traditions:** Establish family traditions that celebrate individual milestones and accomplishments. This can help create lasting memories and reinforce the significance of each child's journey.

2. Encouraging Shared Experiences

Facilitating shared experiences among siblings can enhance their bond and promote understanding.

- **Family Activities:** Engage in family activities that encourage collaboration and teamwork, such as game nights, outdoor adventures, or arts and crafts projects. These experiences foster connection and create lasting memories.
- **Volunteer Together:** Consider engaging in volunteer opportunities as a family. Working together to support others can deepen the bond among siblings and promote empathy.

Building a Supportive Network

Creating a supportive network can be invaluable for siblings of children with special needs. Connecting with others who share similar experiences can help them feel less isolated and provide a platform for sharing.

1. Sibling Support Groups

Sibling support groups provide a safe space for children to connect with others facing similar challenges. These groups can help siblings articulate their feelings and share their experiences.

- **Finding Local Groups:** Research local support groups or online communities that focus on siblings of children with special needs. These groups can provide valuable insights, resources, and a sense of camaraderie.
- **Facilitated Discussions:** Encourage siblings to participate in facilitated discussions within these groups. Sharing their experiences can provide validation and foster understanding.

2. Education and Awareness

Providing siblings with education about their sibling's special needs or disability can foster understanding and compassion.

- **Age-Appropriate Resources:** Seek out age-appropriate books, videos, or workshops that explain the specific challenges and strengths of their sibling's condition. This can enhance empathy and reduce feelings of confusion. One of the best resources for siblings is the **Sibling Support Project** founded by **Don Meyer** in 1990, which is a nationwide community that connects and supports siblings of people with disabilities, offering resources, peer support, and advocacy to strengthen sibling roles across their lifespans. The Sibling Support Project is a partner organization with the national Sibling Leadership Network, which has chapters in twenty-nine states (https://siblingsupport.org).

    Don was also featured in the SFN Dads Zoom Call, Siblings & Family Balance, on July 21, 2020, which can be found on the 21st Century Dads YouTube channel.
- **Family Education:** Consider attending workshops or seminars together as a family to learn more about the unique needs of the

child with a disability or medical condition. Understanding can help siblings feel more connected and supportive.

The Importance of Resilience

Building resilience in siblings is essential for their emotional and social well-being. Resilience can empower children to navigate the challenges they may face, both within the family and beyond.

1. Encouraging Coping Strategies

Teaching siblings effective coping strategies can equip them with tools to manage their emotions and experiences.

- **Mindfulness Techniques:** Introduce mindfulness techniques, such as deep breathing or visualization, to help siblings manage stress and anxiety. These practices can provide a sense of calm and grounding. Practicing daily breathing exercises and yoga have been proven ways to create a sense of centeredness. SFN Mentor Father **Azim Khamisa** is an outspoken advocate for the impact of mindfulness and forgiveness. Very sadly, Azim lost his only son, Tariq, to gun violence at the age of 20.

> *Sustained goodwill creates friendship. Sustained friendship creates empathy. Sustained empathy creates compassion. Sustained compassion creates peace. But people ask me, "How do you extend goodwill to the child who killed your son?" I said, "You do that through forgiveness."*
>
> —**Azim Khamisa**, *Dad To Dad Podcast*, episode #147

- **Problem-Solving Skills:** Encourage siblings to develop problem-solving skills by discussing challenges openly and collaboratively. Empowering them to find solutions fosters confidence and resilience.

2. Fostering Independence

One of the things all parents want for their children is to be self-sufficient and independent. Encouraging independence in siblings can enhance their sense of self and promote personal growth.

- **Allowing Autonomy:** One of the parenting philosophies I embraced early on is not doing for your child what they can do for themselves. Allow siblings to take ownership of their own interests and pursuits. Providing space for individual exploration fosters independence and self-discovery. A great example of this is exemplified in the Carmody family. SFN advocate **Mike Carmody** has witnessed the importance of encouraging siblings to embrace their own path. Mike's brother, John, who has Down syndrome, propelled Mike to create **Opportunity Knocks**, a non-profit on the near west side of Chicago that supports teens and adults with intellectual and developmental disabilities—known in the program as "Warriors"—through dynamic, person-centered, community-based programming. Its core offerings include day, evening, and summer programs focused on life skills, employment readiness, health and wellness, recreation, and community engagement, as well as social enterprise initiatives like the Knockout Kitchen and Knockout Farm that provide real-world vocational experiences while promoting inclusion in the broader community.

> *He's been a guiding force in my life—helping me learn who I am and what I need to do to reach my potential. I think he's helped me truly become the person I'm meant to be.*
>
> *And in turn, I've helped him. I think we've done that together. He's always been my role model.*
>
> —**Mike Carmody,** *Dad To Dad Podcast,* **episode #107**

- **Encouraging Goals:** Support siblings in setting personal goals and working toward them. Celebrating their progress can reinforce their sense of accomplishment and self-worth. Note: The difference between a thought and a goal is that goals are written down.

Doing so helps you clarify what you want to achieve and ensures you are emotionally and intellectually engaged in achieving your goal. The most extreme example I know is with **Warren Rustand**. When Warren, who is 86, was 19, an assignment in a philosophy class was to make a list of the one hundred things he'd like to accomplish in his life. He tells a very compelling story about how laminating that list and looking at it with great frequency propelled him to accomplish ninety-eight of the one hundred items, some of which were quite audacious.

When I was 19 years old, I was in a philosophy class and it just dawned on me that I should probably make a list of the things that I want to do in my lifetime. And so I started writing and I actually listed a hundred items. I still have that list today here, right with me today. And that list is interesting because at 19, there were some things that were kind of soft and squishy on there, and there was some things that were pretty grand.

And so I looked at it about once a week for the next fifty-five or sixty years, actually it's been fifty-nine years since I did that. And I keep that piece of paper enclosed in plastic. It probably would disintegrate because the paper is so old. I looked at it every once in a while. And as a result of looking at it, I tended to accomplish the things that I put on the list.

—Warren Rustand, *Dad To Dad Podcast*, episode #142

Conclusion: Embracing the Sibling Bond

In the journey of parenting a child with special needs, it is vital to recognize and nurture the significance of sibling relationships. Keep in mind, you're a parent to all your children. While the challenges of balancing attention and love across the family may feel daunting, embracing the unique roles of each sibling can create a supportive and loving environment for everyone.

By prioritizing open communication, celebrating individual achievements, and fostering shared experiences, fathers can cultivate strong bonds among siblings, promoting empathy, resilience, and understanding. As siblings learn to navigate the complexities of family dynamics, they often emerge as compassionate individuals who appreciate diversity and embrace the strengths within their family.

Ultimately, the sibling bond is a precious gift that enriches the family experience. In most cases the sibling relationships will endure well beyond our lifetimes. By investing time and love into these relationships, fathers can foster an inclusive environment that empowers all children to thrive—together, as a family.

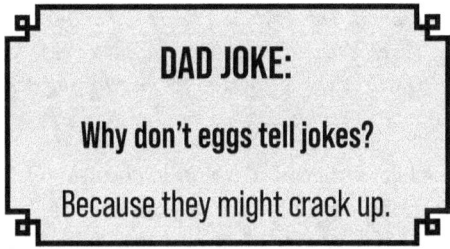

DAD JOKE:

Why don't eggs tell jokes?

Because they might crack up.

- 10 -
Family Leadership: Building a Strong, Healthy, and Unified Household with Vision, Intent, and Values

FATHER AS LEADER

I stand as a pillar, steady and true,
Guiding our home through storms we push through.
Not just by words, but actions I lead,
Planting the roots of love that we need.

My child's not broken—no, they shine bright,
A soul full of courage, a heart full of light.
Together we rise, no mountain too steep,
With faith as our anchor, our bond running deep.

> "Leadership is not about being in charge. It is about taking care of those in your charge."
> —Warren Rustand, SFN Mentor Father and author, *The Leader Within Us*

In the intricate landscape of family life, leadership is not confined to formal roles or titles. It embodies the essence of guiding, nurturing, and cultivating a unified and thriving household. Family leadership is about creating a vision that encompasses the unique needs of each family member, particularly when raising children with special needs. This chapter delves into the principles of family leadership, emphasizing the importance of **vision**, **intent**, and **values** in fostering a strong, healthy, and unified household.

The Concept of Family Leadership

Family leadership transcends traditional notions of authority; it is about creating an environment where every member feels valued, understood, and empowered. It is a dynamic process that involves communication, collaboration, and the cultivation of relationships based on mutual respect and understanding.

1. Embracing Shared Responsibility

In a family, leadership should not rest solely on one parent's shoulders. Instead, it should be a shared responsibility that encourages involvement from all family members.

Collaborative Decision-Making: Encourage family discussions about important decisions. This collaboration fosters a sense of ownership and encourages everyone to contribute their perspectives. One of the most enlightening examples of this was the central message in the interview with **Jen Lumanlan** of Berkeley, California, who is a researcher and founder of **Your Parenting Mojo** and host of a podcast by the same name.

> *I think we've covered a lot of ground. So if there were one thing to leave you with, it's this:* ***needs****. Needs underpin everything.*
>
> *They underpin your child's difficult behavior. They underpin your own mental inflexibility—and why you sometimes can't say yes to something. When we understand needs, we can find strategies that meet both of our needs the vast majority of the time.*
>
> —**Jen Lumanlan,** *Dad To Dad Podcast*, **episode #371**

Rotating Roles: Consider rotating responsibilities for various family tasks or projects, allowing everyone to develop leadership skills and learn the importance of contributing to the household.

2. The Power of Vision

A compelling vision serves as a guiding light for the family, directing decisions and fostering a sense of purpose. Creating a vision involves articulating shared goals, values, and aspirations.

Defining Family Values: Engage in discussions to define your family's core values. These values may include compassion, resilience, love, and acceptance. A shared understanding of these values creates a foundation for decision-making and interactions.

Setting Goals Together: Work together as a family to establish both short-term and long-term goals. Involve everyone in the process, ensuring that each member feels included and that their aspirations are acknowledged.

Intentionality in Family Leadership

Intentionality refers to the conscious effort to align actions with the family's vision and values. Being intentional in family leadership involves making deliberate choices that prioritize the well-being of each family member. The gold standard in this area is having a written family mission statement. Historically this has been the domain of ultra-wealthy families who benefit from the counsel of consultants. A family mission statement has little to do with financial wealth and much to do with the importance about naming important family values and passing them along as part of your legacy.

One of the best examples of this is the Singletary family. My friend Mike Singletary, of the 1985 Super Bowl Champion Chicago Bears football team, is one of the most intentional family men I know. He and his wife, Kim, have seven children. They crafted a family mission statement that was literally posted on an archway in their house for their kids to see and live by every day:

> *This is the Home of Champions—As Singletarys, we will always strive to do our very best in all we do. We will strive to be honest and respect each other's feelings, property, and time. We will always pray for one another, fight for one another, and encourage one another. For our trust be not in our home, nor our money or status or knowledge, but in each other and above all, our Lord and Savior, Jesus Christ.*

Carson and Warren Rustand also have a written family vision statement:

> *An eternally sealed family which helps each member reach their potential through unconditional love, respect for differences, where all are committed to lead Christ-centered lives, and which serves as a protective shield for all within.*

For additional information on creating a family mission statement, scan the QR codes or go to: www.focusonthefamily.com/parenting/writing-a-family-mission-statement/ or www.leaderinme.org/blog/create-family-mission-statement-3-steps

1. Prioritizing Time Together

In the fast-paced world we live in, it can be easy for families to become disconnected. Prioritizing quality time together is a key aspect of intentional family leadership.

Family Rituals: Establish regular family rituals or traditions, such as family game nights, movie nights, or shared meals. These rituals create opportunities for connection and strengthen family bonds. Did you know researchers at the Family Dinner Project found that "over three decades of research have shown that regular family meals offer a wide variety of physical, social-emotional and academic benefits" to children (https://thefamilydinnerproject.org/about-us/benefits-of-family-dinners)? They found kids who live in homes that enjoy regular family dinners are more likely to experience:

- Better academic performance
- Higher self-esteem
- Greater sense of resilience, and
- Much more.

Scheduled Check-Ins: Implement regular family check-ins where each member can share their thoughts, feelings, and experiences. Here are several reasons why establishing this practice can be transformative. Such check-ins can promote open communication, strengthen bonds, encourage emotional awareness, help with conflict resolution, and create lasting memories. For a more comprehensive dive into the value of regular family check-ins, go to https://realitypathing.com/how-to-start-a-weekly-family-check-in-ritual.

2. Encouraging Individual Growth

While unity is essential, it is equally important to recognize and support the individual growth of each family member.

Personal Development Plans: Encourage each family member to set personal goals and pursue their interests. Support their endeavors by providing resources, time, and encouragement.

Celebrating Achievements: Acknowledge and celebrate individual achievements, no matter how small. Recognizing accomplishments fosters self-esteem and reinforces the family's commitment to personal growth.

Values as the Foundation of Family Leadership

Values serve as the bedrock of family leadership, influencing behavior, decision-making, and relationships within the household. By establishing and embodying core values, families can create a culture of respect, love, and support.

1. Modeling Values in Action

As parents and family leaders, it is crucial to model the values you wish to instill in your children. I'm a firm believer that actions speak louder than words. One of the most influential people in my life was my maternal grandfather, Sam Solomon, who became my primary positive adult male role model when my parents divorced. As mentioned previously, we shared a very close relationship. It was my good fortune to be born on his birthday, to be his first grandchild, and to enjoy nearly forty years together. He died in 2001, at age 93. At his funeral, I had the privilege to eulogize him and shared this quote from Ralph Waldo Emerson:

> *"Your actions speak so loudly, I cannot hear what you are saying."*

What values do you want your children and grandchildren to "inherit" from you?

- **Demonstrating Empathy:** Show empathy and understanding in your interactions with each family member. Responding with kindness and compassion sets an example for children to follow.

- **Community Engagement:** Involve your family in community service or volunteer work. Engaging in acts of kindness reinforces values such as compassion and generosity.

One of the reasons I had so much reverence for my Grandpa Sam was his commitment to service. He and his older brother, Joe, sold their business, Solomon Drug Co., in the 1950s, well before I came along. Starting in his late 40s, my grandfather would spend the next forty years as a volunteer pharmacist, as well as serving as a Mason and Shriner.

Looking back, I can see clearly my knowledge of and interest in service was developed at an early age. But it wasn't only my grandfather who had an influence on me.

As I'm writing this passage, we just learned that former US President Jimmy Carter passed away at age 100. If my grandfather was the one who modeled service for me, it was President Carter who put it on steroids. Here's the short story.

In 1990 I was appointed to be the national service project chairman for Theta Xi National Fraternity. I felt then and feel today, that all high school and college-age youth should have a positive service-learning experience. My "job" was encouraging the 2,500 men at more than fifty college campuses across the US to increase their commitment to service. While serving as national service project chairman, I was invited to travel to Liberty City Miami, as one of 350 volunteers, to participate in the Jimmy Carter Work Project. Starting with concrete slabs on Monday morning, our objective was to build ten homes and a day care center, with ribbon-cutting ceremonies planned for Saturday. And that's what we did. In addition to witnessing the power of community coming together on behalf of these ten families, I had another epiphany.

President and Rosalynn Carter were some of the first people on site each morning and some of the last to leave each day. They stood in the same lines we did for our cafeteria-style food and slept in the same unfurnished dorm rooms. For the record, they did have a Secret Service detail present the entire time.

On the flight home, I was reflecting on the experiences and the many transformations that had taken place. The big takeaway for me was thinking, *If the former president of the United States can dedicate a week out of his busy schedule to such service, certainly average people, like me, should be able to do the same.* Every year since, I've dedicated at least one week a year to a cause or causes.

Thank you, Grandpa Sam and Jimmy Carter, for helping me understand and embrace the value of service.

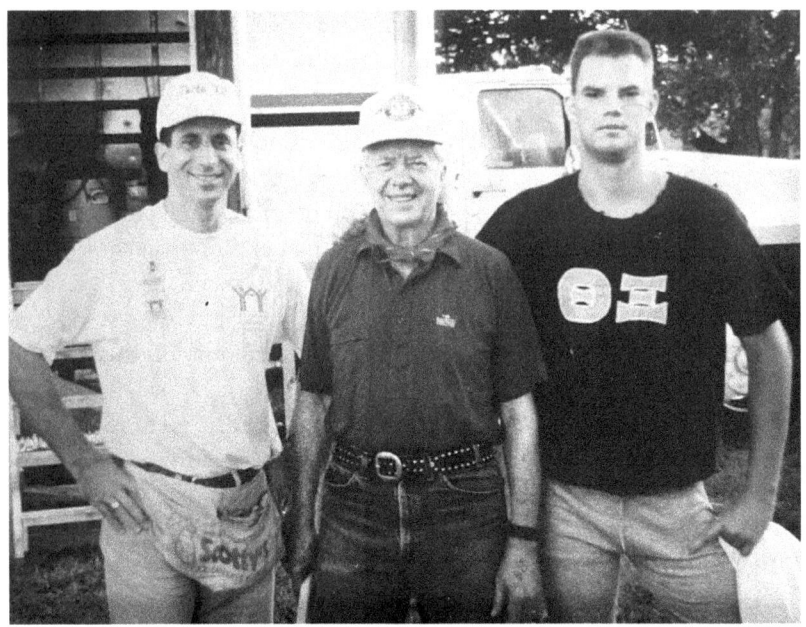

From left: David, former US President Jimmy Carter, and Frank McSweeney

2. Creating a Value-Driven Environment

Building a value-driven environment requires consistent reinforcement and integration of values into daily life.

- **Value Statements:** Create value statements that articulate your family's core beliefs. Display these statements prominently in your home as reminders of the principles you and your family strive to uphold.
- **Discussing Values:** Regularly engage in discussions about your family's values and their relevance to everyday situations. Encourage children to share their interpretations and experiences related to these values. A prime example of this took place in the interview with **Warren Rustand**.

When you become a teenager, you grow out of certain things. You're expected to have better behavior in lots of ways, be smarter, all that kind of stuff. And so those conversations are really elevated conversations about who are you? And where are you going? And what are you doing? And what did you do today? What did you read today? What did you think about today?

> *Parents can be their advocates or they can use inquiry. You can use advocacy or inquiry. And you can use both.* ***Advocacy*** *is really this notion of you're telling people what to do. You're commanding people what to do. You have a stated position. A stated view.* ***Inquiry*** *is really where we think most of parenting is done. And that's asking questions and allowing children to critically analyze their answers and responses and think things through and come to their own conclusions.*
>
> —Warren Rustand, *Dad To Dad Podcast*, episode #142

Communication: The Cornerstone of Family Leadership

Effective communication is the cornerstone of successful family leadership. Open and honest communication fosters understanding, reduces conflict, and strengthens relationships.

1. Encouraging Open Dialogue

Creating an environment where family members feel comfortable expressing their thoughts and feelings is crucial for healthy communication.

- **Active Listening:** Practice active listening by giving full attention to each family member when they speak. Validate their feelings and demonstrate empathy in your responses. Active listening is a learned communication practice. Active listening involves mastering a whole host of other skills—from learning how to read subtle cues to controlling your own emotional response. It requires both empathy and self-awareness. **Amy Gallo** wrote an excellent column for *Harvard Business Review* on active listening. As she explains, it builds trust, reduces misunderstandings, and makes others feel genuinely heard—leading to stronger relationships and better outcomes.
- **Creating Safe Spaces:** Establish safe spaces for family discussions, where everyone feels secure in sharing their thoughts without judgment. This can be as simple as a designated time during family meals or dedicated family meetings. As mentioned previously, family mealtimes are an essential ingredient to creating and maintaining consistent quality family time and for sharing life.

2. Navigating Difficult Conversations

Addressing challenging topics, such as the needs of the child with the disability or significant health condition, requires sensitivity and openness.

- **Approaching Conversations with Care:** When discussing difficult subjects, approach the conversation with care and empathy. Be mindful of each family member's feelings and perspective.
- **Problem-Solving Together:** Engage the family in problem-solving discussions. Encourage each member to contribute ideas and collaborate on finding solutions, reinforcing the importance of teamwork. One expert in this field is **Jonathan Bennett** of Ontario, Canada, a seasoned business professional who now does executive coaching. Jonathan is also the author of seven books. When he and his wife, Wendy, learned their autistic child identified as nonbinary, it tested the family to collaborate and identify a win-win path.

The most important thing I can share with any parent—and especially a parent of an autistic child—is this: The people with the best advice are autistic adults.

Not scientists. Not doctors. Not occupational therapists, physical therapists, or speech-language pathologists—or anyone else. If you really want to understand what's happening in the mind of your child, listen to autistic adults.

—Jonathan Bennett, *Dad To Dad Podcast*, episode #301

Nurturing Resilience Through Leadership

Leadership in the family context also involves fostering resilience among family members. Resilience is the ability to adapt, persevere, and thrive despite challenges.

1. Teaching Coping Strategies

Providing family members with coping strategies equips them with the tools to navigate adversity effectively.

- **Encouraging Expression:** Encourage open expression of emotions, allowing family members to share their feelings during challenging times. This practice normalizes vulnerability and promotes emotional well-being.
- **Promoting Problem-Solving Skills:** Teach children how to approach challenges with a problem-solving mindset. Encourage them to brainstorm solutions and evaluate potential outcomes collaboratively. Are you familiar with the "Ben Franklin approach"? Very simply stated, this approach is a structured pros-and-cons decision method. Franklin recommended drawing a line down a sheet of paper, listing the pros on one side and the cons on the other, and then weighing each item by its relative importance. Once the pros and cons are lined up, side by side, the right decision becomes more obvious.

2. Embracing a Growth Mindset

Cultivating a growth mindset encourages family members to view challenges as opportunities for growth and learning.

- **Reframing Challenges:** Encourage family members to reframe challenges as learning experiences. Celebrate efforts and progress rather than solely focusing on outcomes. In an effort to get my kids to look at both sides of a situation, one of my go-to questions has been "Is that a positive or a negative situation?"
- **Sharing Stories of Resilience:** Share stories of resilience within the family, whether from personal experiences or external examples. Highlighting resilience reinforces the idea that overcoming challenges is a shared journey. One example that comes to mind is **Randy Pierce** of Concord, New Hampshire. In his early 20s Randy suddenly went blind in one eye and then, over several years, lost sight in the other eye. If that wasn't challenging enough, Randy also lost the ability to walk for the better part of two years. After a series of medical procedures and through old-fashioned grit and determination, Randy regained his ability to walk and has become an avid outdoorsman and mountain climber, including summiting Mount Kilimanjaro in Tanzania.

> *We're all distinctive. And that uniqueness is where our strengths come from.*
>
> *You're going to have a strength that I may not. And I might have one you don't. Imagine if we shared those strengths so we could both benefit—and vice versa.*
>
> —**Randy Pierce,** *Dad To Dad Podcast*, **episode #388**

Building Unity in Diversity

In families with children who have special needs, unity can be further enriched by celebrating diversity. Embracing the unique qualities of each family member contributes to a more robust family dynamic.

1. Acknowledging Individual Strengths

Recognizing and celebrating the unique strengths and contributions of each family member fosters a sense of belonging and appreciation.

- **Strength-Based Discussions:** Hold family discussions focused on individual strengths. Encourage each member to share what they believe makes them unique and valuable to the family.
- **Leveraging Strengths for Teamwork:** Utilize each member's strengths in family activities or projects. This collaboration promotes teamwork and reinforces the importance of diverse contributions.

2. Celebrating Family Differences

Diversity within the family should be celebrated, as it enriches the family experience and fosters a culture of acceptance.

- **Embracing Unique Perspectives:** Encourage family members to share their unique perspectives and experiences. These discussions can promote empathy and broaden everyone's understanding.
- **Family Traditions That Embrace Diversity:** Create family traditions that celebrate diversity, whether through cultural celebrations, unique family rituals, or shared hobbies that reflect each member's interests.

The Role of Family Leadership in Times of Crisis

In times of crisis or significant challenges, effective family leadership becomes even more critical. During such periods, families need strong leaders to navigate uncertainty and provide support.

When I think about family leadership and crisis, the Goldberg-Polin family comes to mind. On October 7, 2023, Hersh Goldberg-Polin, 23 years old, was among the 240 hostages taken by the Palestinian militant group Hamas during its attack on Israel. I had the privilege of interviewing **Jon Polin**, Hersh's dad, on August 30, 2024, on Hersh's 328th day of his captivity. To that point, his mother, Rachel Goldberg-Polin, and Jon had displayed an unparalleled level of strength and courage, vocally advocating for the release of Hersh and the remaining roughly 100 living hostages. As a result, the family was thrust into the limelight, meeting with members of the United Nations in Geneva, Switzerland and Pope Francis in Rome, as well as then-US President Joe Biden. Then the week before our interview, the two appeared on stage at the Democratic National Convention in Chicago on August 21, pleading for the release of all the hostages.

Tragically, just days after the interview was recorded and two days before the interview aired, the world learned that the Israel Defense Forces had recovered the bodies of six hostages, including Hersh, who had been mercilessly executed within the previous twenty-four to forty-eight hours.

On September 2, while eulogizing Hersh at his funeral, Jon said:

> *We have received such an outpouring of love, strength, support, and prayers from people literally all over the world—every day—for 328 days. We get messages from people on every continent. And we know that we're not alone in this mission.*
>
> *I mentioned earlier that I grew up playing sports. There's something about this mission where, every day that passes, we have more and more people supporting us. It feels like if we don't get up every morning and spring out of bed to hit the day and do everything we can for these hostages, not only are we failing ourselves and Hersh—but we're letting our team down.*
>
> —**Jon Polin,** *Dad To Dad Podcast***, episode #337**

1. Leading with Compassion

Compassionate leadership involves understanding the emotional toll that challenges can take on each family member.

- **Being Present:** During difficult times, ensure that you are present for each family member, offering emotional support and encouragement. Your presence can be a stabilizing force amid uncertainty.
- **Creating a Safe Space for Emotions:** Foster an environment where family members feel safe expressing their fears and concerns. Encourage them to share their feelings openly, allowing for emotional processing. One technique for doing this is sharing your emotion and then asking your child to share theirs. This is particularly important with your boys, since girls are often socialized to be more open in sharing their emotions.

2. Navigating Change Together

Change can be unsettling for families, especially when it involves a child with special needs. Leading through change requires collaboration and adaptability.

- **Establishing Routines:** During periods of change, establish routines that provide structure and predictability for family members. Consistent routines can help alleviate anxiety and promote a sense of stability.
- **Adapting Together:** Encourage family members to adapt to changes together, reinforcing the idea that challenges are best navigated as a team. Emphasize flexibility and open-mindedness in approaching new circumstances.

Conclusion: Empowering Family Leadership

Family leadership is an evolving process that requires intentionality, communication, and a commitment to fostering unity and resilience. By embracing shared responsibility, articulating a compelling vision, and nurturing the values that define your family, you can create a strong, healthy, and unified household.

As you navigate the complexities of family life, remember that leadership is about serving those in your charge—your children, your partner, and yourself. By prioritizing their needs, fostering open communication, and celebrating the unique strengths of each family member, you lay the foundation for a thriving family dynamic.

Embrace the journey of family leadership with purpose and love, for it is through your guidance that each family member can flourish and reach their full potential. The lessons learned and the bonds formed through family leadership will resonate for generations to come, creating a legacy of love, resilience, and unity.

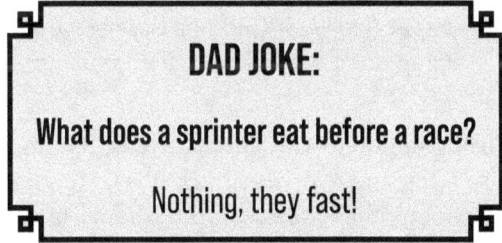

DAD JOKE:

What does a sprinter eat before a race?

Nothing, they fast!

- 11 -
Mastermind Groups: Tapping into Collective Wisdom and Support

GUIDED STRENGTH

In a circle of minds, I find my way,
Voices of wisdom help light my day.
No path alone, no burden solo,
Lessons shared make courage grow.

A father's love, both fierce and true,
Yet stronger still with a broader view.
Through trials deep, through endless flight,
Masterminds turn dark to light.

"The only way to succeed is to have people around you who want to see you succeed."
—Aaron Walker, founder of Iron Sharpens Iron, a brotherhood designed specifically for Christian business leaders, owners, and entrepreneurs, and host of the *Iron Sharpens Iron Podcast*

As fathers raising children with special needs, the journey can sometimes feel isolating and overwhelming. Navigating medical appointments, educational challenges, and emotional ups and downs can take a toll on both mental and physical well-being. One effective way to combat this isolation is through mastermind groups, where fathers gather weekly to share experiences, seek advice, and build a supportive network.

This chapter will explore the concept of mastermind groups, highlighting their benefits, structure, and the commitment required to participate effectively. Additionally, we'll discuss the importance of annual in-person retreats to deepen connections and foster growth.

Understanding Mastermind Groups

A mastermind group is a gathering of like-minded individuals who come together to support one another in their personal and professional growth. The concept, popularized by Napoleon Hill in his book *Think and Grow Rich*, is rooted in the idea that the collective wisdom and experience of a group can lead to greater success for everyone.

1. The Essence of Mastermind Groups

Mastermind groups are built on collaboration and mutual support. Each member contributes their unique insights, experiences, and expertise in a safe and nurturing environment.

- **Collective Intelligence:** The combined knowledge of a group can provide innovative solutions to common challenges faced by fathers of children with special needs. Discussions can lead to new perspectives and insights that might not emerge in isolation.
- **Support and Accountability:** Members hold each other accountable for their goals and commitments. This accountability fosters motivation and encourages individuals to stay on track, promoting personal growth and progress.

2. Benefits of Joining a Mastermind Group

Participating in a mastermind group can offer numerous advantages, particularly for fathers raising children with special needs. Here are some key benefits:

- **Emotional Support:** Mastermind groups provide a safe space for fathers to share their feelings and experiences. Connecting with others who understand the unique challenges can alleviate feelings of isolation and stress.
- **Resource Sharing:** Members often share valuable resources, tips, and strategies that can help address common challenges. This sharing of information can save time and provide actionable insights.
- **Networking Opportunities:** Mastermind groups facilitate connections with other fathers who may have similar experiences or expertise. These connections can lead to collaborations, friendships, and valuable networking opportunities.
- **Safe and Nurturing Environment:** Most men do not have a place they feel safe to be open and authentic. While some actively search for such a place, most men aren't aware that such a place exists. In

other words, you don't know what you don't know. Do yourself a favor and take the plunge and join or help start a group. It may just transform your life, the way it has for so many others.

The Structure of a Mastermind Group

To ensure that meetings are productive and focused, mastermind groups typically follow a structured format. Here are common elements that contribute to the success of these gatherings:

1. Meeting Frequency and Duration

The most successful mastermind groups meet on a weekly basis. Meeting less frequently has proven not to achieve the same results and leads to attrition.

- **Weekly Virtual Meetings:** With the rise of technology, weekly virtual meetings have become increasingly popular. They allow members to connect from the comfort of their home or office, eliminating travel time and costs, accommodating busy schedules, and providing valuable support.
- **Time Commitment:** Members should agree on a set duration for each meeting, typically ranging from one to two hours. This time frame allows for in-depth discussions while respecting everyone's time constraints.
- **Leadership:** Meetings are led by a different group member each week. The group leader and Dad in the Middle are included in the master calendar created at the beginning of the year. Dads know weeks and months in advance when they are leading the meeting and when they are scheduled to be a Dad in the Middle.

2. Meeting Agenda

Having a clear agenda helps keep meetings focused and productive. Here's a typical structure for a 75-minute weekly SFN Mastermind Group meeting:

- **The First 15 Minutes:** We start each meeting with a brief round of "wins" from the past week. Each member shares wins, large and small, since the last meeting.
- **The Second 15 Minutes:** We read six books a year. Each week we typically discuss one or two chapters of the current book.

Members are asked to read, reflect, and resolve to incorporate a takeaway from the experience. On preassigned dates, six times a year, we have a Zoom call with the author to discuss their book and have an intimate conversation. This is just one of many things that makes the mastermind group experience so special. (For a full list of all the books read and reviewed since July 2021 until February 2026, see Appendix A.)

- **The Next 30 Minutes:** This time is where one member at a time presents a challenge he is facing and seeks input and support from the group. These challenges might have to do with their atypical child, their typical child or children, their marriage, or issues with their health, with family members, or at work. This focused attention allows for deep problem-solving and brainstorming.
- **The Last 15 Minutes:** The remaining time is dedicated to what each member is looking forward to in the week ahead. This time is also used to share resources, goal setting, and accountability. This practice reinforces accountability and ensures that members leave with actionable steps. To reiterate, we start and end each SFN Mastermind Group weekly meeting on a positive note.
- **One Final Thought:** These weekly SFN Mastermind Group meetings are no place to play the hardship Olympics. While we tackle some very difficult situations, these are not gripe sessions.

Time and Financial Commitment

Participating in a mastermind group requires both time and a financial commitment. Understanding these aspects is crucial for ensuring a successful experience.

1. Time Commitment

While the time commitment for each meeting may seem manageable, it's essential to consider the overall time investment.

- **Preparation:** Members should allocate suitable time to prepare for each meeting. In most cases this means staying current with any reading requirements. Members give some advanced thought to the "win(s)" from the past week. If you're the Dad in the Middle, you will need to think about the issue or challenge you're wrestling with and want to discuss.

- **Ongoing Participation:** Consistency and active participation are key to reaping the benefits of a mastermind group. Members should prioritize attendance and engage fully in discussions, making the most of the collective wisdom available. The old adage that "what you get out of something is in direct proportion to the time you invest" definitely applies to one's participation in mastermind groups. Dads do occasionally miss meetings due to last-minute schedule conflicts, health issues, and travel challenges.
- **Statement of Intent:** SFN Mastermind Group Dads sign an annual Statement of Intent, which lists the principles they agree to adhere to, including attending weekly meetings, respecting the opinions of others, and honoring the confidentiality of members, to name a few. (See Appendix A for the full SFN Mastermind Group Statement of Intent.)

2. Financial Commitment

Historically, mastermind groups have been composed of business leaders seeking revenue growth, advice from like-minded peers, personal development, and camaraderie. The most successful and longest-lasting mastermind groups all involve a financial commitment, to cover the costs of resources, annual and semiannual meetings, and administration. Each person in the fifteen mastermind groups that are part of Aaron Walker's Iron Sharpens Iron Mastermind Groups make a $500–$700 monthly commitment.

As a result of our friendship and Aaron's commitment to supporting the Special Fathers Network, he donated the *ISI Mastermind Playbook* to the 21st Century Dads Foundation. 21CD branded its mastermind program as the SFN Mastermind Group and utilizes a dynamic pricing model.

- **Monthly Commitment:** The SFN Mastermind Group commitment is $200 per month, or whatever each member can afford (minimum of $50 per month). This dynamic pricing model has allowed younger dads and those without higher-paying jobs to participate. The financial commitment each dad makes is confidential, which means everyone has an equal seat at the table. Regarding the financial commitment, most dads would say that their family is the most important aspect of their lives. Whether a dad makes $50,000 a year, $150,000 a year, or substantially more, making a $600 or more commitment per year is a small investment

to make to get plugged into a group of like-minded dads committed to being present physically, emotionally, and spiritually for one another.
- **Shared Resources:** What does the $50–$200 per month cover? In addition to the actual out-of-pocket costs of books, journals, and administrative expenses, the monthly commitment also covers the annual in-person retreat, including hotels, meals, and local excursions.

Annual In-Person Retreats

While virtual meetings are valuable, annual in-person retreats take the mastermind experience to a new level. Retreats provide opportunities for deeper connections, focused discussions, and collaborative problem-solving. While the COVID-19 pandemic increased the popularity of virtual meetings, nothing can replace the experience of being physically present and having shared experiences.

1. The Value of In-Person Connections

In-person retreats foster a sense of camaraderie that can be difficult to achieve through virtual meetings alone. Spending time together in a relaxed setting allows members to build deeper relationships, leading to enhanced trust and open communication. In-person retreats provide a dedicated time and space for focused discussions and brainstorming. The absence of daily distractions allows for deeper engagement and creativity.

2. Planning Successful Retreats

To maximize the benefits of an annual retreat, careful planning is essential. Here are some key considerations:

- **Choosing a Location:** Select a location that is convenient and conducive to group activities. The annual SFN Mastermind Group Retreats have been hotel-based in centrally located cities, including Nashville, Tennessee, St. Louis, Missouri, and Chicago, Illinois.
- **Creating an Agenda:** Developing a retreat agenda is a balancing act that includes structured discussions, workshops, and opportunities for informal networking, plus some downtime for relaxation as well as informal conversations.

- **Incorporating Guest Speakers:** Including guest speakers is a sure way to generate some energy and make the overall experience more meaningful and memorable. Speakers can provide fresh perspectives and inspire new ideas. Here is a list of the locations of the SFN Mastermind Group Retreats and the featured guest speakers:
    - **2021:** Nashville—Aaron Walker, serial entrepreneur, founder of Iron Sharpens Iron, and author of *View from the Top*.
    - **2022:** St. Louis—Scott Newport of Royal Oak, Michigan, a retired craftsman, gifted communicator, and SFN Mentor Father.

> *We can't do this alone. We need other dads around us. We need our families, our wives, the pastors at the church, and Children's Special Health Care. We need our social workers. We need the teachers. I can't do this alone.*
>
> **—Scott Newport,** *Dad To Dad Podcast,* **episode #179**

- **2023:** Chicago—my dear, longtime friend Tom Dreesen, stand-up comedian who opened for Frank Sinatra for thirteen years, speaker, and author of *Tim & Tom: An America Comedy in Black and White*.

> *And as we were running to the limo, a woman started screaming, "Mr. Sinatra, please—Mr. Sinatra, please!"*
>
> *Frank got out of the limo and went up to her. "What is it, ma'am?"*
>
> *She said, "My husband is home sick—terribly ill. If I could get an autograph from you, it would mean the world to him."*
>
> *Frank said, "Sure." He signed an autograph and handed it to her.*
>
> *She said, "Oh, what beautiful cuff links." They were very expensive—over a thousand dollars.*
>
> *When he finished signing, he took off the cuff links and handed them to her, saying, "Give these to your husband."*

She said, "No, no, no—I don't want them. I was just admiring them."

He said, "No. I want your husband to have them."

—**Tom Dreesen,** *Dad To Dad Podcast,* **episode #250**

- **2024:** Chicago—Wayne Messmer, serial entrepreneur, singer, speaker, and author of *The Voice of Victory: One Man's Journey to Freedom Through Healing and Forgiveness.*

A 15-year-old ran up on me. Never heard him, never said a word, never heard him coming. And the first two sounds were him banging on the window, right next to my ear on the driver's door. So bang, bang, boom, and as I hit the gas to pull out, boom, he pulls the trigger. Nine-millimeter shot point-blank in the neck. Oy. What do you do? What do you do? What do you do? What do you do? You survive. I, I grab onto life. Okay, what do I do?

—**Wayne Messmer,** *Dad To Dad Podcast,* **episode #56**

- **2025:** Chicago—Randy Lewis, former executive vice president at Walgreens, author, TEDx speaker, and one of the most well-respected advocates for employment for the disability community.

We said, "When we do this, if we're successful, we're going to give it away. We're going to open our doors to the world, even our competitors."

And I think that appealed to people that we were working for something bigger than us. And I think that has challenged everybody and inspired everybody to do it. So they set a goal for a thousand, achieved it, and then they set a goal for two thousand, 20 percent, which they're working on now. And we did give away. So lots of other companies came. Best Buy. P&G came. UPS. Companies overseas. Marks & Spencer in the UK. And it continues to grow.

—**Randy Lewis,** *Dad To Dad Podcast,* **episode #2**

Creating and Maintaining a Successful Mastermind Group

In lieu of joining one of the existing SFN Mastermind Groups, consider starting one yourself. It's as simple as:

1. Identifying Potential Members

Choosing the right members is crucial for the success of your mastermind group. Look for individuals who share similar values, goals, and experiences. While shared experiences are important, diversity in backgrounds, expertise, and perspectives can enrich discussions. Seek out members with various skill sets and experiences to foster deeper insights. Leverage existing networks, social media, or local support groups to identify potential members. Reach out to other fathers who may benefit from a supportive community.

2. Setting Group Guidelines

Establishing clear guidelines helps create a structured and respectful environment for discussions. Use the SFN Mastermind Group Statement of Intent found in Appendix A.

3. Selecting Meeting Platforms

Choosing the right platform for virtual meetings is crucial for smooth communication and engagement. Utilize user-friendly video conferencing tools such as Zoom, Google Meet, or Microsoft Teams. Familiarize all members with the chosen platform to ensure seamless participation. Consider setting up a group chat platform (e.g., by text or utilizing WhatsApp) for ongoing communication, resource sharing, and accountability between meetings.

Best Practices for Effective Mastermind Meetings

To maximize the benefits of your mastermind group, consider implementing the following best practices during meetings:

1. Be Prepared

Preparation is key to productive discussions. Encourage members to come to meetings with specific topics or challenges they would like to address. After each meeting, remind members to follow up on action items discussed. Accountability is strengthened when members report back on their progress during subsequent meetings. We created the

SFN Mastermind Group journal for this purpose so dads can take notes week to week in an organized fashion.

2. Foster Engagement

Encourage active participation from all members to create a dynamic and supportive atmosphere. Encourage members to ask questions and provide feedback during the Dad in the Middle segments. This engagement fosters collaboration and deeper understanding. Rotating the leadership role for each meeting is one of the keys, allowing each member to hone skills in facilitating discussions. This practice empowers members and promotes shared ownership of the group.

Overcoming Challenges in Mastermind Groups

While mastermind groups can be incredibly rewarding, they may also face challenges. Here are some common obstacles and strategies for overcoming them:

1. Managing Different Commitment Levels

Differences in commitment levels among members can lead to frustration or disengagement. Establish regular check-ins to assess members' engagement and commitment levels. Openly discuss any concerns and encourage accountability. Recognize that life circumstances may impact members' availability. Be open to flexible participation, allowing members to contribute in ways that suit their current situations.

2. Navigating Conflict

Disagreements or conflicts may arise within the group, particularly when discussing sensitive topics. Create guidelines for navigating conflict constructively. Encourage open dialogue and promote understanding among members. Remind members of the group's shared goals and aspirations, redirecting discussions toward constructive solutions. When I was a young businessperson, my maternal grandfather coached me to avoid talking about religion and politics. While not a mastermind group taboo, steering away from divisive issues helps maintain group harmony.

Conclusion: The Power of Collective Wisdom

Mastermind groups offer a powerful avenue for fathers navigating the complexities of raising children with special needs. By tapping into collective wisdom and support, fathers can access valuable resources, emotional encouragement, and actionable insights to enhance their parenting journey.

As you embark on the journey of creating or participating in a mastermind group, remember the words of Aaron Walker: *"The only way to succeed is to have people around you who want to see you succeed."* Being part of a community of fathers who share similar experiences can and will change the trajectory of your life. Surrounding yourself with like-minded individuals fosters an environment of support, accountability, and growth.

Embrace the power of collaboration and collective wisdom as you navigate the challenges of fatherhood. By investing time and effort in the relationships of a mastermind group, you can cultivate meaningful connections that enrich not only your life but also the lives of your family members. Together, you can thrive in the beautiful, complex journey of parenting children with special needs.

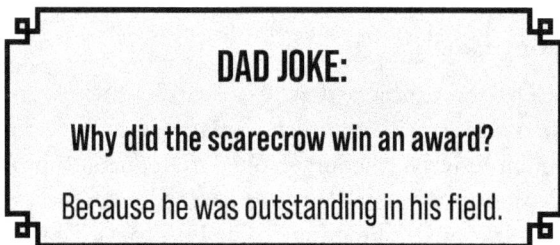

DAD JOKE:

Why did the scarecrow win an award?

Because he was outstanding in his field.

- 12 -
IEPs, Setting and Accomplishing Goals, and Celebrating Wins, Large and Small

THE LANGUAGE OF LOVE

You do not speak the way they do,
Yet every glance, I hear what's true.
A touch, a smile, a soft embrace,
Your love is written on your face.

No words are needed, not a sound,
To know our bond is deep, profound.
And though the world may fail to see,
Your voice is clear—it speaks to me.

"Every small victory is a stepping stone to greater achievements. Celebrate every success, no matter how small."
—John Crowley, chief executive officer,
Biotechnology Innovation Organization (BIO)

In the journey of fatherhood, particularly when raising children with special needs, it can be easy to become consumed by the challenges and hurdles that often accompany daily life. The demands of medical appointments, therapy sessions, and educational advocacy can overshadow the many achievements, both big and small, that deserve recognition. This chapter tackles the world of IEPs (Individualized Education Programs), setting and accomplishing goals, and emphasizes the importance of celebrating these wins.

As fathers, we often find ourselves navigating unfamiliar systems, challenging assumptions, and learning new languages of care, education, and support. Among the most influential tools a family encounters along this path is the IEP. But as meaningful as the IEP can be, it represents only one part of a much larger story—a story of goals, growth, resilience, and the importance of celebrating wins both big and small.

Over the years, the *SFN Dad To Dad Podcast* has featured numerous guests who have lived deeply inside this journey. Their reflections—whether as parents, educators, advocates, or a combination of the above—offer fathers a clear message: The IEP is important, but it is not the whole picture. True growth comes from setting meaningful goals inside and outside of school, staying attuned to progress wherever it occurs, and celebrating the moments that remind us that our children are becoming exactly who they are meant to be.

IEPs—A Foundation, Not a Finish Line

For many dads, the IEP is the first major intersection between parenting and advocacy. It often marks the moment when a father realizes just how much his presence matters. Walking into an IEP meeting—whether the first or the fifteenth—can feel intimidating. The table may be filled with specialists offering assessments, recommendations, and technical language that can overwhelm even the most confident parent. Yet this is also the place where a dad's voice carries tremendous weight.

Catherine Whitcher, a master IEP coach and a professional non-attorney advocate, emphasizes that the IEP is most effective when parents are active participants rather than silent observers. Dads do not need to be experts; they simply need to bring what only they as a parent can offer—deep insight into their child's strengths, motivations, and lived experience. The educational team sees the child in a structured environment. Parents see the child in life. When both perspectives come together, the plan improves.

> *Every family is so different. Every child's path is so different. And educators do not know the inner workings of your family. But if you share it with them and you collaborate with them, they can design a program that not only supports a child at school, but supports them for a lifetime.*
>
> —**Catherine Whitcher**, *Dad To Dad Podcast*, episode #202

Louis Geigerman, an advocate, spent years supporting families who felt overwhelmed by the process. He consistently observed that when fathers engaged—whether by asking questions, offering context, or sharing what works at home—the team's understanding of the child expanded. His experience reinforces a simple but powerful truth: A present father can help humanize the process.

> *Everything I believed regarding my son came from what I observed—because I knew him better than anybody else. And that's something parents really need to understand. You'll have all these experts come in and start giving opinions and advice. But don't ever forget: You are the person who knows your child better than anyone else. Don't ever forget that.*
>
> —**Louis Geigerman**, *Dad To Dad Podcast*, **episode #177**

Still, creating the IEP is not always easy. Sometimes disagreements arise. Services fall short. Goals don't align with parental expectations. **Jim Rigg**, who is superintendent of Catholic Education for the Archdiocese of Miami, is also the parent of a child with autism. He has chosen to educate his child in public schools. He reminds us that navigating the IEP process can be emotionally challenging even for seasoned educational professionals when they find themselves as the parent at the IEP table. That feeling is normal. What matters is staying engaged and remembering that the IEP is not static; it is revisited, revised, and refined as the child grows.

> *I've seen that most schools, with a little bit of open-mindedness, flexibility, and compassion—and a willingness to do things differently—can accomplish a lot.*
>
> *You don't always need a full-time aide or a new wing built onto your school to serve a child with special needs. You can do a lot with just an open mind and a little flexibility and compassion.*
>
> —**Jim Rigg**, *Dad To Dad Podcast*, **episode #73**

IEP teams also benefit from a strength-based mindset, something **DeAndrae Hinton**, an educator in Texas, and **Patrick Schwarz**, a highly respected education consultant, each emphasized from their own professional perspectives as educators. When the conversation focuses on what the child can do—as opposed to what they cannot—teams become more creative, hopeful, and solution-oriented. Strengths open doors. Strengths inspire new pathways. And strengths remind everyone at the table that the purpose of the plan is not to limit a child, but to elevate them.

> *I was on a mission to find the strengths in every person I came across with autism or another disability. I'd say, "I know there's a superpower in you somewhere."*
>
> *Once people understood that I was genuinely on a mission to find their strengths and help them, you started to see a real change. You saw them appreciate school more. You saw them begin to believe in themselves.*
>
> —DeAndrae Hinton, *Dad To Dad Podcast*, episode #355

> *Oftentimes, if you can tap into someone's gifts and talents, you can find ways to strategically support their areas of struggle or disability.*
>
> *That's an example of turning disability into possibility.*
>
> —Dr. Patrick Schwarz, *Dad To Dad Podcast*, episode #376

Ultimately, the IEP provides a foundation: a structured document where goals, supports, and expectations are written down and agreed upon. But it is only the beginning. Unfortunately, families often find the IEP isn't being followed and may have to advocate for more accountability.

Setting and Accomplishing Goals Outside the IEP

While the IEP sets official goals within the educational system, fathers quickly discover that their child's development extends far beyond the school walls. In some ways, the most important goals are the ones designed and nurtured at home—goals that arise from a child's interests, from daily routines, or from the desire to build independence, confidence, and resilience.

Goal setting begins with understanding who your child is. Strengths, passions, challenges, and rhythms all matter. For some children, goals may focus on communication, emotional regulation, or social engagement. For others, they may involve mobility, life skills, or academic enrichment. What matters most is that the goals are meaningful, achievable, and relevant to your child's world.

Guests like Catherine Whitcher and DeAndrae Hinton emphasize the importance of tying goals to real life. A reading goal might be connected to following a recipe. A math goal might emerge from budgeting for a family outing. A physical goal might weave naturally into play, movement, or chores. Fathers often discover that goals are not separate from life at all—they *live* in life.

Accomplishing goals is rarely linear. Children move at their own pace. They may leap ahead one week and stall the next. What matters is consistency, patience, and adaptability. Fathers become guides who help shape the environment, create opportunities, and scaffold experiences so that their child can succeed. Sometimes this happens intentionally, through structured practice or targeted support. Other times it happens spontaneously with a teachable moment during a walk, a conversation in the car, a shared task in the kitchen.

SFN guests frequently describe how important it is for fathers to view progress broadly. A goal does not need to be large to be significant. A child initiating a simple request, managing frustration, staying engaged in an activity, or helping with a household task may signal enormous development. When dads recognize these moments, they help reinforce learning and build momentum.

Goal accomplishment is not just about skill development; it can also be about identity. A child who meets goals—no matter how modest—may begin to see themselves as capable, more competent, and worthy of pride. That shift in self-perception becomes the fuel for future growth.

And fathers, more than anyone else, help anchor this sense of capability.

Celebrating Wins—Large and Small

If the IEP provides structure and goal setting provides direction, then celebration provides purpose. Celebration is what infuses the journey with hope. It is what helps families endure the slow, uneven progress that characterizes so much of special needs parenting. It is also one of the most powerful tools a father can offer his child.

Celebrating wins does not always come naturally. Many dads become so focused on what needs improvement—on what isn't working, what skills remain unmastered, what barriers remain—that they forget to acknowledge the tremendous effort being made every single day. But progress in the special needs world is often measured in inches, not miles. And those inches matter.

When a child sees that their efforts are recognized, their confidence grows. When a father pauses to acknowledge a small step—a new sound, a gesture, a moment of calm, an act of kindness, or a spark of independence—he communicates something essential: *I see you, and I am proud of you.*

Celebrations need not be elaborate. In fact, the most meaningful ones often occur quietly: a smile at the dinner table, a gentle high-five, a warm acknowledgment during bedtime, or a shared moment of joy after a small accomplishment. Children notice these moments. They carry them. They return to them when things feel hard.

Of course, there are also big wins—significant breakthroughs, important milestones, and achievements that once felt out of reach. These deserve their own rituals. A family outing. A favorite treat. A phone call to a grandparent. A photo or journal entry to cement the moment in memory. Fathers often discover that celebrating big wins anchors gratitude and grounds the family in hope.

Yet the greatest impact comes from recognizing the daily victories— the ones no one else sees. The brave effort a child makes to try again. The resilience they show after a setback. The quiet patience during a stressful moment. These wins shape character, resilience, and identity. And when fathers make a habit of noticing and celebrating them, they transform the entire journey.

Conclusion: A Father's Steady Hand

The IEP may provide a formal structure, goals may serve as guideposts, but celebrations—especially celebrations rooted in a father's attention and love—are the heartbeat of the journey.

Through hundreds of SFN conversations, a clear truth emerges: Children thrive when their fathers recognize their effort, believe in their potential, and celebrate their progress. A father's steady encouragement and hope can dramatically enhance the educational plans, therapy schedules, and intervention strategies.

In the end, navigating IEPs, setting meaningful goals, and celebrating wins are not just tasks—they are expressions of love. They say to a child: *I am with you. I see you. I believe in you. And I am here for every step—especially the small ones.*

And those small steps, celebrated faithfully, often lead to the biggest transformations of all.

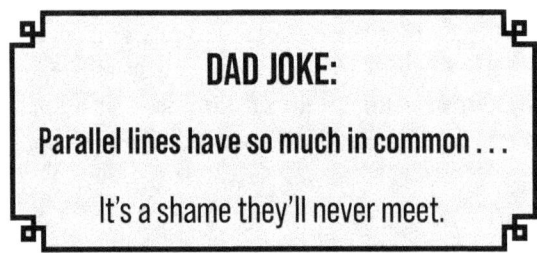

- 13 -
Living in the Present: Thriving in the Circumstances You Didn't Expect

EMBRACING TODAY

The path's not straight, the road's not clear,
Yet love outshines the weight of fear.
A child's laugh, a hand in mine,
Teaches me that now is fine.

Plans may shift, the storms may rise,
But joy still sparks in tired eyes.
Not what I dreamed, yet more than gold—
A story rich, a heart made bold.

"Many times we spend our lives waiting for the circumstances to change, forgetting that we have the power to change our perspective."
—Noel Fernández Collot, author of *Vivir según las circunstancias* (*Living According to the Circumstances: A Memoir*), an 82-year-old retired Baptist pastor in Cuba, featured in episode #317 of the *SFN Dad To Dad Podcast*

Fathers raising children with special needs often find themselves navigating uncharted waters. The road can be filled with unexpected challenges, twists, and turns that can leave dads feeling overwhelmed, uncertain, exhausted both physically and mentally, as well as anxious about the future. However, in these moments of unpredictability, fathers are presented with a unique opportunity to cultivate resilience, embrace the present, and thrive in the circumstances most never anticipated.

In this chapter, we explore the importance of living in the present, practical strategies to foster mindfulness, and ways to cultivate a positive outlook amid life's uncertainties. By doing so, we can create a fulfilling environment for ourselves and our families, one where we not only adapt to our circumstances but thrive within them.

The Importance of Living in the Present

Living in the present is about acknowledging our current reality rather than fixating on the past or worrying about the future. It encourages us to engage fully with our experiences and to appreciate the moments that make up our daily lives.

1. Acceptance of Reality

When faced with unexpected circumstances, acceptance is the first step toward finding peace. Accepting our current situation does not mean resignation; rather, it involves acknowledging the reality of our lives without judgment. **Example:** If a child is diagnosed with a special need, acceptance means recognizing that this is now part of your family's story. Instead of being in denial or dwelling on the "what ifs" or the life you had envisioned, you can focus on creating a new narrative that includes the strengths and joys of your child. There is a famous 1987 poem entitled "Welcome to Holland" by **Emily Perl Kinsley**, which beautifully lays out the importance about accepting the alternative path and embracing the circumstances. While not applicable to all families, many parents can relate to the message.

To read the full poem, go to:
https://www.emilyperlkingsley.com/welcome-to-holland
or scan the QR code.

2. Reducing Anxiety

By concentrating on the present, we can reduce anxiety associated with uncertainty about the future. While it's healthy to think and plan for the future, worrying about what might happen can lead to stress and cause us to feel overwhelmed, while living in the moment allows us to experience life as it unfolds. Mindfulness practices, such as deep breathing, meditation, and grounding exercises, can help anchor us in the present moment, allowing us to let go of worries and create a sense of calm.

3. Cultivating Gratitude

Living in the present helps us cultivate gratitude for the moments we often take for granted. By shifting our focus from what is lacking to what is available, we can find joy and appreciation in everyday experiences.

Keeping a gratitude journal where you record moments of gratitude each day can reinforce a positive mindset. This simple practice can transform our perspective and encourage us to seek out the beauty in our circumstances. I started keeping a gratitude journal after completing the RCIA program in the spring of 2011, at age 50. Each night before going to sleep, I jot down the five to ten things that I'm thankful for that occurred during the day. The journal also doubles for where I record my prayer requests. While I have very rarely ever gone back and read these journal entries, by doing this before going to bed, it has helped train my mind to plant these seeds of gratitude shortly before I transition from conscious to unconsciousness, every night.

Practical Strategies for Thriving in the Present

To thrive in the circumstances we didn't expect, it's essential to implement practical strategies that promote mindfulness, acceptance, and positivity. Here are several approaches to consider:

Practice Mindfulness. Mindfulness is the practice of being fully present and aware of our thoughts, feelings, and sensations without judgment. It encourages us to immerse ourselves in the current moment rather than getting lost in worries or regrets.

- **Mindful Breathing:** Take a few minutes each day to focus on your breath. Inhale deeply through your nose, hold for a moment, and exhale slowly through your mouth. This practice can ground you in the present and calm racing thoughts.
- **Mindful Listening:** During conversations with your child or partner, practice mindful listening by fully engaging in the dialogue. Focus on their words, tone, and emotions rather than formulating your response. This practice enhances connection and strengthens relationships.

Set Realistic Goals. Setting realistic goals can help you navigate unexpected circumstances while fostering a sense of purpose. Goals should be achievable and aligned with your current situation.

- **Short-Term Goals:** Break down larger objectives into smaller, manageable steps. For example, if your child is working on communication skills, set a goal for them to learn a new word each week. Celebrate each small achievement as a win.
- **Adjust Expectations:** Be flexible with your goals and expectations. Understand that progress may look different than you initially envisioned. Adapt to your child's pace and celebrate each step forward. Patience is the primary virtue here. One of the best examples of this is the 1% Better Every Day program utilized by SFN Mentor Father Nik Nikic, of Maitland, Florida, whose son Chris, was the first person with Down syndrome—on the planet—to complete the full Ironman distance triathlon: swimming 2.4 miles in open water, biking 112 miles, and running 26.2 miles. What Nik learned is that Chris is capable, but it takes him much longer to accomplish milestones than typical athletes.

Coincidentally I was also competing in my second Ironman triathlon in November 2020, and I witnessed Chris's historic accomplishment. There were dozens and dozens of supporters along the sidelines, wearing neon-colored 1% Better T-shirts, cheering on Chris. It was a palpable experience.

> *One day I said, "We're going to change." And I started telling everybody around him, "I need you to stop treating my son like he has special needs. I need you to treat him like he's special—like he's gifted."*
>
> *And lo and behold, look what he's done. In the last six months, he's become something of a global celebrity. He's accomplished things nobody ever thought were possible. He has speaking engagements. People from different places are sponsoring him. It's amazing what he's accomplished once we started to believe he was gifted—and we let him pursue that gift.*
>
> —Nik Nikic, *Dad To Dad Podcast*, episode #108

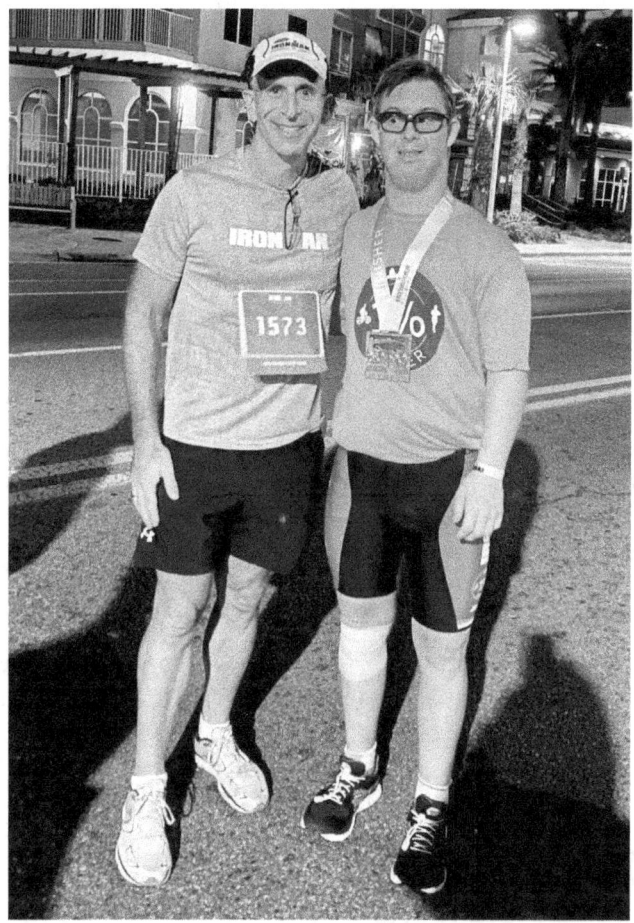

David and Chris Nikic after the Ironman Florida triathlon in November 2020

Embrace Flexibility. Flexibility is essential when navigating the unpredictable nature of raising children and especially a child with special needs. Being open to change or pivoting allows us to respond positively to new challenges and opportunities.

- **Adapt Plans:** If an outing or planned activity doesn't go as expected, be willing to adjust your plans. Instead of feeling frustrated, try to find joy in the unexpected moments that may arise.
- **Practice Letting Go:** Release the need for control and embrace spontaneity. Often, the most memorable experiences come from unplanned moments that arise when we let go of rigid expectations.

Who hasn't been at a restaurant, a store, or a friend's house when a child (yours or someone else's) has a meltdown or acts inappropriately? **Lon Haldeman**, an SFN Mentor Father from Sharon, Wisconsin, shared a profound insight. Since tragically losing his daughter Erica to juvenile ALS at 11 months of age, Lon views children acting up, while out at dinner or in public, differently, and we should too.

You have to look on the bright side and make the best of it. You can't just dwell on the negative—that would be overwhelming.

The way we handled it with Erica was to keep her involved in our lives— traveling across the country with us. You have to try to stay optimistic, even in Erica's case, when there really wasn't much hope. That was probably the hardest part—knowing how predictable the outcome was likely to be.

—Lon Haldeman, *Dad To Dad Podcast*, episode #124

Focus on Strengths. Shift your focus from challenges to the strengths of your child and family. First, understand the medical model, which is a mainstream perspective of disability, is based on deficits. There is a baseline or typical level of physical and intellectual development, usually based on age, and anyone who is below that threshold is considered deficient. As an example, consider the world of IEPs. To qualify for IEP resources, a student must have a deficit and a qualifying educational disability that adversely affects their educational performance. The implied objective is to reduce that gap or to get a child to the "age-appropriate" grade level.

While the benefit of focusing on the deficit is your child qualifies for extra services and is entitled to certain accommodations, the unintended consequence is this a glass-half-empty way of looking at the situation. An alternative is to look at the same situation and focus instead on what is working and what is possible. Celebrating strengths fosters a positive environment that encourages growth and resilience.

Highlight Achievements. Regularly acknowledge and celebrate your child's achievements, regardless of how small they may seem. This practice reinforces their sense of capability and encourages them to continue striving for success.

Identify Family Strengths. Take time as a family to identify and discuss your unique strengths. Recognizing what each family member brings to the table fosters appreciation and unity.

Build a Support Network. Surrounding yourself with a supportive community can help you navigate the challenges of unexpected circumstances. Building relationships with other fathers and families can provide valuable insights, resources, and encouragement.

- **Join Support Groups:** Look for local or online support groups for fathers of children with special needs. Connecting with others who share similar experiences can alleviate feelings of isolation and provide a sense of camaraderie.
- **Engage in Community Activities:** Participate in community events or activities that promote connection and support. Building relationships within your community fosters a sense of belonging and provides a network to lean on during tough times. Here is a partial list of community-based activities and events to consider:
    - **Inclusive Playground Days.** Visit playgrounds designed to be accessible for children of all abilities. Many communities have inclusive play spaces. If there is no such playground in your community, consider helping create one.
    - **Adaptive Sports Leagues.** Join sports programs such as baseball, swimming, or soccer that accommodate children with special needs. Keep in mind that Special Olympics is for those with intellectual disabilities, while adaptive sports are for those with physical disabilities.
    - **Sensory-Friendly Movie Screenings.** Attend movie screenings tailored to children with sensory sensitivities, often offered by local theaters.
    - **Art and Music Therapy Workshops.** Participate in art and music classes specifically designed for children with special needs and their families.
    - **Local Library Storytime.** Many libraries host sensory-friendly story times with adjustments for different needs.
    - **Community Festivals.** Check for events with quiet zones or accommodations for families with special needs.
    - **Adaptive Dance or Movement Classes.** Enroll in dance or movement programs that focus on inclusivity and adaptation for various abilities.

- **Therapeutic Horseback Riding.** Explore equine therapy programs, which can be both therapeutic and enjoyable for children with disabilities.
- **Outdoor Nature Walks.** Visit nature trails or parks that are wheelchair-accessible and provide a calm environment for family exploration.
- **Special Needs Parent Support Groups with Family Activities.** Join a group that hosts events for the whole family, offering fun activities while connecting with other parents. For example, Joni and Friends, the global Christian disability ministry, offers week-long family retreats.

For more information, go to:
https://joniandfriends.org/family-retreat/
or scan the QR code.

Navigating Grief and Acceptance

Unexpected circumstances often come with feelings of grief and loss, particularly regarding the life we had envisioned for our families. Navigating this grief is a crucial part of the journey toward acceptance and thriving in the present.

Acknowledge Grief. Recognizing and accepting feelings of grief is essential for healing. It's normal to grieve the life you anticipated, and acknowledging these emotions can be a powerful step toward acceptance.

- **Express Emotions:** Allow yourself to express your feelings, whether through journaling, talking with a trusted friend, or engaging in creative outlets. Processing emotions can help you find clarity and understanding.
- **Seek Professional Support:** If feelings of grief become overwhelming, consider seeking support from a therapist or counselor. Professional guidance can provide valuable tools and insights for navigating these emotions. My observation is that a majority of seasoned and well-adjusted special needs dads have sought out professional help. Somehow, someway they have been able to buck the innate male tendency to "figure out things on our own."

Find Meaning in the Journey. Reframing your perspective to find meaning in your experiences can help you move forward. Instead of focusing solely on what you've lost, look for opportunities for growth and connection.

- **Explore New Interests:** Discover new interests and hobbies that align with your current circumstances. Engaging in activities that bring joy and fulfillment can help shift your focus from loss to growth.

> *I'm having to heal physically. I'm having to heal spiritually, and for me to heal, the best way is to serve others and to give, not to focus on myself.*
>
> —Dr. Stephen "Doc" Hunsley, *Dad To Dad Podcast*, episode #122

Embracing Hope

Hope is a powerful force that can propel us forward, even in the face of uncertainty. By cultivating hope, we can inspire ourselves and our families to thrive amid unexpected circumstances. Hope can thrive in some of the most unlikely circumstances, as it did for SFN Mentor Father **Tim Kuck** of Bell Isle, Florida, father of three, including Nathaniel, born in June 1997 and who passed away in 2001, at age 4, as the result of multiple birth anomalies, including duodenal atresia and craniosynostosis. Tim and his wife, Marie, redirected their grief into creating **Nathaniel's Hope**, a nonprofit organization that provides free respite care, birthday parties, and other programs for children with special needs and their families. Nathaniel's Hope positively impacts more than ten thousand families annually.

> *There was a nurse standing over my son's bed, and she said, "There's something about this boy. There's just something about this boy. Can I pray for you?"*
>
> *And we were like, "You know, we're kind of spiritually bankrupt—emotionally bankrupt—trying to care for our son." So she prayed for us. But she didn't pray that he would be healed and go home. She prayed that his **purpose** would be fulfilled.*

> *I remember thinking, **what an odd prayer** for this little boy who doesn't walk, or talk, or eat with his mouth. It felt prophetic—like foreshadowing.*
>
> *And that's exactly what we believe.*
>
> —Tim Kuck, Dad To Dad Podcast, episode #57

Practice Positive Affirmations. Affirmations are positive statements that can help reshape our mindset and reinforce hope. Incorporate affirmations into your daily routine to foster a positive outlook.

- **Daily Affirmations:** Create a list of affirmations that resonate with you and your family. Repeat these affirmations daily to remind yourself of your strength, resilience, and capacity for growth. Take it a step further and post the list of affirmations in highly visible places like the bathroom mirror, in the kitchen, or next to your computer.
- **Encourage Children:** Teach your children to use positive affirmations to boost their confidence and self-esteem. Encourage them to create their own affirmations that reflect their strengths and abilities.

Celebrate Progress. Regularly celebrating progress, no matter how small, can help maintain a hopeful outlook. Acknowledging growth reinforces the belief that positive change is possible.

- **Create a Progress Chart:** Develop a visual chart to track progress toward goals or milestones. Celebrate each step achieved, reinforcing a sense of accomplishment and hope.
- **Reflect on Growth:** Take time to reflect on how far you and your family have come. Acknowledge the challenges faced and the resilience shown, reinforcing a narrative of growth and hope. Consider saving short videos in an album on your phone that can be played back a year or years down the road.

Conclusion: Thriving in Uncertainty

As Noel Fernández Collot wisely stated, *"Many times we spend our lives waiting for the circumstances to change, forgetting that we have the power to change our perspective."* Living in the present allows us to embrace our reality, foster resilience, and thrive amid the circumstances we didn't expect.

By implementing practical strategies such as mindfulness, flexibility, and community support, we can navigate the challenges of fatherhood with grace and strength. Acknowledging our grief and finding meaning in our experiences allows us to build a hopeful narrative for ourselves and our families.

As you embark on this journey, remember that you have the power to create a fulfilling and meaningful life, even in the face of uncertainty. Embrace the present, celebrate the victories, and thrive in the beautiful complexity of your family's journey. Together, you can create a supportive, loving environment where everyone can flourish, regardless of the circumstances that life presents.

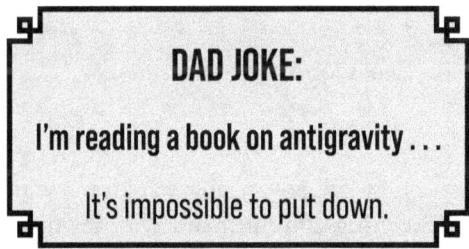

- 14 -
The Unwavering Commitment: 24/7/365 Fatherhood and What It Really Takes

24/7/365

Through sleepless nights and weary days,
I walk beside you, come what may.
Not just in moments, bright and few,
But every breath—I'm here for you.

Through every triumph, tear, and test,
I give my all, I give my best.
Not part-time love, nor fleeting ties,
But steadfast hands and watchful eyes.

24/7, rain or shine,
Every heartbeat, yours and mine.
Through each challenge, high or steep,
A father's promise—strong and deep.

"Life is too short to be ordinary."

—Dick Hoyt

Fatherhood, especially when raising children with special needs, demands an unwavering commitment. It is not merely a role we fulfill during specific hours or days; it is a profound commitment that requires us to be present, engaged, and resilient 24 hours a day, 7 days a week, 365 days a year. This chapter explores what it means to embrace fatherhood in its entirety, reflecting on the dedication required, the challenges faced, and the profound rewards that come from this journey.

The Nature of Unwavering Commitment

Unwavering commitment in fatherhood involves a dedication that goes beyond conventional parenting responsibilities. It encompasses emotional, physical, and mental engagement that shapes the well-being of both the father and the child.

Understanding the Depth of Commitment. Commitment as a father means being there for your child not just in moments of triumph but also during challenges, setbacks, and everyday routines. This type of dedication requires recognizing that fatherhood is a marathon, not a sprint. **Example:** Whether it's waking up in the middle of the night for a child's needs or being an advocate during school meetings, commitment involves showing up consistently, regardless of the circumstances. In some situations, it requires making sacrifices and putting our own needs or wants aside.

Building a Foundation of Trust. An unwavering commitment fosters a foundation of trust between fathers and their children. Children thrive in an environment where they know their fathers will always be there for them, no matter what. Trust building means regularly showing up for your child, engaging in *their* interests, and being available for conversations. Building such trust can positively influence their emotional and social development.

Embracing the 24/7/365 Commitment

Being a dedicated father means being available around the clock, not just during times of need but also during everyday moments of joy and growth.

The Everyday Commitment. Fatherhood encompasses countless small yet significant moments that contribute to the overall well-being of the child. These moments create lasting memories and foster strong bonds.

- **Daily Routines**: Engaging in daily activities, such as preparing meals, doing chores together, and sharing bedtime stories, reinforces the commitment to being present in your child's life.
- **Education:** Research from the US Department of Education documents that when both parents are involved in their child's education, educational outcomes go up and many of the issues which hold kids back—and that are some of society's greatest challenges, such as crime and incarceration, drug and alcohol use,

and teen suicide and pregnancy—go down. Here are some ways to demonstrate your commitment to your child's education:

- Read to your child.
- Review your child's homework.
- Attend parent-teacher conferences and IEP meetings.
- Know each of your child's teachers by name.
- Volunteer at your child's school.
- Create a healthy home environment for academic work.
- Review your child's report cards and IEP progress reports.

- **Active Participation:** Being involved in your child's routines, therapy sessions, and activities not only supports their development but also strengthens your connection as a father.

Balancing Responsibilities. Commitment often requires balancing various responsibilities, including work, family obligations, and self-care. This balance is crucial for sustaining long-term engagement in fatherhood. When I think about balance, SFN Mentor Father **Rick Daynes** of San Diego, California, comes to mind. Rick is the father of five, including three with special needs: one with Down syndrome, one with autism, and one with what was then called Asperger's syndrome, now simply diagnosed as autism spectrum disorder. Rick is also the author of *Keep It Together Man: For Dads with a Special Kid*.

> *He saw it, ran over, and got the trophy. And I'm telling you—after all the garbage we'd gone through, all the things we tried to get him involved in, all the times we took him out of the house to walk or go to the beach hoping something would click—all of that suddenly felt validated.*
>
> *Because he stood there on the podium with his trophy. I looked at my wife, and she was just bawling. Tears flowing. It was maybe the happiest moment we'd had in years.*
>
> —Rick Daynes, *Dad To Dad Podcast*, episode #45

- **Time Management:** Developing effective time management skills can help fathers prioritize their commitments. Creating a schedule that allocates time for family, work, and self-care is essential for maintaining balance. Think of these three as legs to a

stool: Each is necessary for stability. Extending the stool analogy, consider the importance of adding a fourth leg to the stool and including spirituality. Adding that fourth dimension can provide even more stability.
- **Shared Responsibilities:** Involving partners or support systems can alleviate the pressures of fatherhood. Think of this as dividing and conquering. Sharing responsibilities with your spouse, family members, and hired help ensures that the commitment to your child is upheld, while also allowing for self-care or some personal time.

The Mental and Emotional Toll

The commitment to fatherhood, particularly in challenging circumstances, can take a toll on mental and emotional well-being. It's critically important to recognize these challenges and develop coping strategies.

Recognizing the Stressors. Raising a child with special needs can be rewarding but can also bring unique stressors, including financial burdens, emotional strain, and societal pressures.

Identifying Stressors: Take time to identify specific stressors that affect your mental and emotional health. Understanding these challenges allows you to address them proactively. Here is a starter list of known stressors:
- **Financial Pressures:** The cost of specialized therapies, treatments, and education, as well as limited work opportunities due to caregiving responsibilities.
- **Emotional Strain:** Coping with the initial diagnosis and long-term implications, along with the fear and worry about your child's future and independence.
- **Relationship Challenges:** Strain on marital or coparenting relationships due to differing coping mechanisms, as well as difficulty balancing time between your partner, your other children, and the child with special needs.
- **Social Isolation:** Feeling misunderstood or judged by others and concerns about job security due to frequent time off for appointments or emergencies.
- **Physical Exhaustion:** Long hours providing care, often leading to sleep deprivation, plus managing medical needs or physical care that can be physically demanding.

- **Lack of Support:** Limited access to resources, support groups, or community services; feeling like you need to handle everything yourself.
- **Educational Advocacy:** Navigating the complexities of IEPs, ensuring that your child receives appropriate accommodations, or frustration with school systems or untrained educators.
- **Sibling Dynamics:** Balancing the needs of your other children in the family, who may feel overlooked, while managing sibling relationships and fostering understanding.
- **Future Uncertainty:** Worrying about what will happen to your child when you are no longer able to provide care, as well as concerns about establishing long-term financial and caregiving plans.

Coping Strategies. Developing healthy coping mechanisms is essential for managing stress and maintaining overall well-being. Here is a partial list of coping strategies:

- **Self-Care Practices:** Incorporating self-care practices, such as exercise, meditation, or hobbies, can provide necessary breaks and rejuvenation. Taking care of yourself enables you to be present and engaged with your child.
- **Support Networks:** Building a network of fellow fathers or joining support groups can provide a space to share experiences, seek advice, and receive encouragement. Connecting with others facing similar challenges helps reduce feelings of isolation. These can be both virtual as well as traditional face-to-face experiences.
- **Seek Professional Help:** Engage with therapists, counselors, or family therapists to address anxiety or emotional challenges. Connect with special education consultants or case managers to navigate services and resources for your child.
- **Learn About Your Child's Condition:** Educate yourself about your child's diagnosis to better understand their needs and advocate effectively, as well as stay informed about therapies, tools, and strategies that can enhance your child's development.
- **Communicate Openly:** Maintain open, honest communication with your partner and family members to share the emotional and practical load, as well as regularly checking in on each other's mental well-being and divide responsibilities.

- **Focus on Abilities, Not Disabilities:** Celebrate your child's strengths, achievements, and unique qualities as well as shift the narrative from challenges to potential growth and opportunities.
- **Plan for the Future:** Establish financial and legal plans (e.g., special needs trusts, wills) to ensure long-term care and security for your child. Consult financial advisors and attorneys who specialize in families with special needs. One SFN Mentor Father to consider is **Chris Hunter** of Orlando, Florida, who has dedicated his practice to serving families touched by disability.

> *Everything good in my life has come into my life through her. You notice a pattern here?*
>
> *She was teaching autistic children to swim, and she came to me and said, "Chris, you have to find a way to help these people. These parents are on an island, and they don't know what to do. I don't care what you do—but if you do anything, do this for me."*
>
> *And that was almost thirty years ago.*
>
> —Chris Hunter, *Dad To Dad Podcast*, episode #345

- **Set Realistic Expectations:** Avoid comparing your child's progress to others, set achievable, individualized goals, and be willing to acknowledge that not every challenge will have an immediate solution.
- **Engage in Advocacy:** Advocate for your child's needs in educational, health-care, or community settings. Being proactive can provide you with a sense of control and purpose.
- **Take Breaks and Delegate:** Accept help from family, friends, or respite care services when offered. Taking time for yourself prevents burnout and enhances your ability to care for your child effectively.

The Power of Resilience

Resilience is a critical component of unwavering commitment. As fathers, we must learn to adapt to adversity, overcome obstacles, and remain steadfast in our dedication.

Embracing Challenges. Rather than viewing challenges as setbacks, fathers should embrace them as opportunities for growth and learning. Challenges can provide valuable lessons that enhance parenting skills.

- **Growth Mindset:** Cultivating a growth mindset allows fathers to approach difficulties with curiosity and resilience. This mindset encourages exploration, adaptation, and finding creative solutions to obstacles. Here are some suggestions:
    - **Practice Self-Reflection:** Regularly reflect on your thoughts, attitudes, and actions. Ask yourself what you've learned from setbacks and how you can improve moving forward.
    - **Celebrate Small Wins:** Focus on incremental progress and celebrate every milestone, no matter how small, to reinforce positivity and perseverance.
    - **Cultivate Patience and Resilience:** Understand that growth is a process. Patience in facing challenges allows for meaningful change and adaptation over time.
    - **Foster a Positive Narrative:** Reframe setbacks as learning experiences and avoid negative self-talk. Focus on what you and your child *can* do, rather than what might seem limiting.
    - **Encourage Effort over Outcome:** Model and teach the value of effort, persistence, and learning through mistakes, which can help both you and your child develop a growth-oriented outlook.
    - **Build a Team of Allies:** Collaborate with your partner, educators, therapists, and other professionals who can support your child's development. Shared resources and teamwork strengthen your capacity to grow.

Celebrating Resilience. Acknowledge and celebrate the resilience demonstrated in both you and your child. Recognizing the strength that comes from facing challenges together fosters a positive outlook and reinforces the commitment to persevere.

- **Resilience Rituals:** Create family rituals that honor resilience, such as sharing stories of overcoming challenges during family gatherings or creating a "resilience wall" showcasing achievements and milestones. Consider these ideas:
    - **Weekly Check-Ins with Partner:** Establish a weekly ritual to connect with your partner, discuss challenges, and celebrate

successes. Open communication builds emotional support and teamwork.
- **Family Gratitude Practice:** Create a ritual where family members share one thing they're grateful for each day. This helps shift focus from challenges to appreciation and fosters a positive family dynamic.
- **Regular Physical Activity:** Engage in consistent physical activities like walking, running, yoga, or weightlifting. Physical movement reduces stress, boosts mood, and builds resilience.
- **Daily Reflection Time:** Dedicate ten to fifteen minutes daily to reflect on positive moments or progress, no matter how small. Journaling or meditating on these moments can provide clarity and gratitude.

Never Giving Up. The essence of unwavering commitment lies in the mindset of never giving up. As fathers, we must embody determination and perseverance, regardless of the challenges that arise. When I think about individuals who are superhuman in their will to persevere, names like David Goggins, a former Navy SEAL and ultra-endurance athlete, and **Bonner Paddock** come to mind. Bonner Paddock of San Diego, California, is the first person with cerebral palsy to complete the Ironman distance triathlon as well as to summit Mount Kilimanjaro. Bonner is also founder of Project Possible, whose mission is to raise awareness and support centers that provide services to empower children with disabilities and their families to live life beyond limits in their communities.

> *Love your child for where they're at. See the beauty in exactly who they are. That is a beautiful, special person who's been gifted into your life, and it's up to you to figure out what those gifts are—each day.*
>
> *See the beauty in them, because there will be great challenges. I know that. I understand the divorce rate is higher. I know there are many challenges that come with raising a child with disabilities.*
>
> *But do your best to love yourself—and to love your loved ones—right where they are.*
>
> —Bonner Paddock, *Dad To Dad Podcast*, episode #230

Finding Inspirational Role Models. Looking to role models can provide inspiration and motivation to embrace the commitment of fatherhood wholeheartedly. Figures such as **Dick Hoyt,** who famously participated in one thousand, two hundred running events, including more than one hundred marathons and six Ironman triathlons, with his son, Rick, exemplify the spirit of never giving up. Dick and Rick faced numerous challenges, yet Dick's dedication to ensuring his son could participate in sports served as a testament to unwavering commitment. Their story serves as a reminder that love and determination can overcome obstacles. Their motto "Yes You Can" is one we can all embrace.

> *And that was in 1981. So we lined up behind the wheelchairs, and we ran. And now, I don't know if you've heard about marathon runners talking about hitting the wall. Well, I hit the wall at twenty-two miles, and I felt terrible. I didn't think I was going to be able to finish it.*
>
> *All the other runners were going by us, and they pounded me on my back and everything else. But we ended up finishing our first marathon in three hours and eighteen minutes, and beat 85 percent of all the other runners.*
>
> —Dick Hoyt, *Dad To Dad Podcast*, **episode #11**

Finding Strength in Adversity. Each challenge faced can serve as an opportunity for growth. Embracing adversity fosters resilience and reinforces the importance of persistence. It's important to do some personal reflection. Take time to reflect on past challenges and identify the strengths developed through those experiences. Acknowledging personal growth reinforces the belief that perseverance pays off.

The Role of Community

The journey of fatherhood is not one that needs to be traveled alone. Building a supportive community can enhance the commitment to raising children—especially a child with special needs.

Building Relationships. Establishing relationships with other fathers can provide invaluable support and encouragement. Sharing experiences and resources fosters a sense of camaraderie and understanding. The power of networking is undervalued. Attend support groups, workshops, or community events focused on special needs parenting. Engaging with others creates connections that can offer guidance and insights. These interactions can be virtual and face-to-face. Dads living in urban areas have more opportunities to interact face-to-face, while dads living in rural areas may find it easier to connect virtually with other special needs dads.

Advocating for Change. Being part of a community allows fathers to advocate for change and raise awareness about the challenges faced by families with special needs. Get involved in local initiatives that support families with special needs. Volunteering or participating in advocacy efforts can create positive change while building connections with others who share similar goals.

Conclusion: A Legacy of Love and Commitment

Unwavering commitment in fatherhood means embracing the journey wholeheartedly, navigating challenges with resilience, and fostering an environment of love and support.

By embodying this commitment 24/7/365, fathers can create a lasting impact on their children's lives and build a legacy of love, strength, and resilience. As you reflect on your commitment to fatherhood, remember the words of Dick Hoyt: *"Life is too short to be ordinary."*

On the face of the Great Dads Coin is the number 247365, which serves as a daily reminder about the ongoing commitment it takes to be a great dad. I carry mine with me every day and everywhere I go. Do you have a Great Dad Coin?

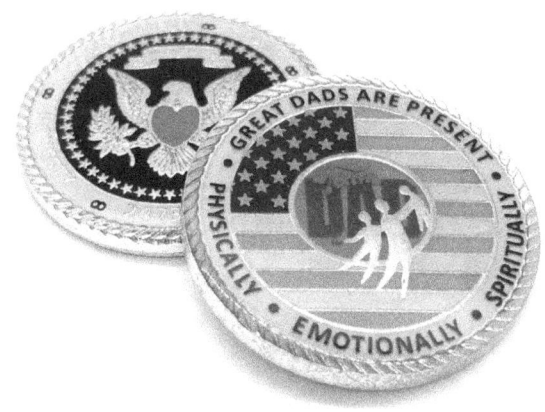

Embrace the extraordinary nature of your journey as a father, never give up, and find strength in the unwavering love you provide. Your dedication is a powerful force that shapes not only your child's future but also the fabric of your family's legacy. Together, you can navigate the challenges and celebrate the triumphs, ensuring that love and commitment remain at the heart of your family's journey.

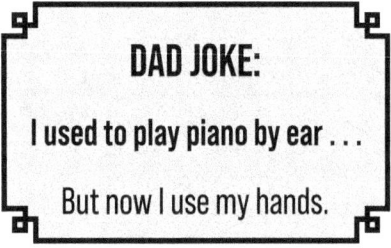

- 15 -
Fostering Independence and Self-Sufficiency: Helping Your Child Build Confidence, Find Purpose, and Gain Employment

STRONG & INDEPENDENT

I guide, not hold, your hand so tight,
You shine so bold, your own true light.
Each step you take, though small, is grand,
I stand with pride, but not command.

Through trials faced, you rise, you grow,
Your strength is more than you may know.
With love, with trust, I step aside,
You soar, my child, with wings so wide.

"People need to be encouraged to think for themselves. It's not about teaching them what to think, but how to think."
—Temple Grandin

"Everybody has a talent, and that talent has to be identified and nurtured. If you can do that, you can change the world."
—Mark X. Cronin

"Successful businesses have to have a diverse workforce that reflects the community."
—Randy Lewis

When you're raising a child with special needs or disabilities, the word *independence* can feel complicated. For some dads, it sounds unrealistic. For others, it feels threatening—almost like independence means our children won't need us anymore. Over the years, I've come to see it very differently.

Independence isn't about doing everything alone. It's about helping our sons and daughters gain as much control over their own lives as possible. It's about making choices, solving problems, contributing to their communities, and, when possible, earning a paycheck or building a business. It's less about separation and more about dignity.

As fathers, we have a unique role in this process. We're often the ones pushing a little, challenging a little, and quietly saying, "I know this is hard, but I also know you can handle more than you think."

"Never Do for a Child What They Can Do for Themselves"

One of my core parenting philosophies has been simple: **Never do for a child what they can do for themselves.** When our kids were young and playing hockey, the equipment bags were almost as big as they were. It would have been faster and easier for my wife or me to carry the bags to and from the rink. But we told them, "If you want to be a hockey player, you carry your own equipment." While they struggled at first, they figured it out.

It wasn't about being harsh. It was about sending a message: *You're capable. This is your sport, your responsibility, your life.*

On the *SFN Dad To Dad Podcast*, I've heard countless versions of this same lesson. One of the most memorable came from my friend **Dan Marquardt**, a father of ten, seven of whom are adopted. Dan described their family dinner with their newly adopted son Kevin, who had come from a very difficult and different cultural background.

> *We're at home, at the dinner table, having our first celebratory "welcome home" dinner with Kevin. I'm feeding him, and Jennifer looks at me and says, "Give him a fork."*
>
> *I said, "He doesn't have any hands." Kevin is our only child who has no hands—and he also has no left foot. But he's an amazing kid.*
>
> *So I got a fork and gave it to Kevin. He looks at the fork. He looks at his siblings and sees how they're all eating. Then he puts his arms together, grabs the fork, flips it over, sticks the food, puts it right into his mouth, and starts feeding himself.*

> *My jaw almost hit the floor. Oh my gosh—it was such a moment.*
>
> *Jennifer, being the amazing mom she is, was immediately in tune with it. It was just instinctive. She said, "Give him a fork." And she was right.*
>
> —Dan Marquardt, *Dad To Dad Podcast*, **episode #15**

Independence usually starts with small, ordinary things, such as carrying your own bag, helping with dinner, learning to tie your shoes, handling a chore without reminders. These tasks build competence. Competence builds confidence. And confidence becomes the engine that drives greater independence.

Building Confidence One Experience at a Time

For most of our children—especially those with disabilities—confidence is not a luxury; it's a necessity. A child who believes "I can figure this out" is far more likely to try, fail, adjust, and try again. A child who has only experienced adults stepping in and doing things *for* them often learns a very different message: *This is too hard for me. Somebody else will fix it.*

That's why it's so important to invite our kids into real responsibilities. Maybe that means helping cook a simple meal, sorting laundry, feeding a pet, or managing a small allowance. At first these tasks might require visual schedules, reminders, or step-by-step prompts. That's okay. The goal is progress, not perfection.

Over time, we can gradually fade our support. Maybe we still check in, but we don't hover. Maybe we let our kids experience the natural consequences of forgetting something or doing a task halfway—and then help them think through how to do better next time. Every time they complete a task, solve a small problem, or recover from a mistake, they're building emotional resilience along with practical skills.

Problem-Solving, Decision-Making, and Self-Advocacy

Independence requires more than technical skills; it requires the ability to process information. Our kids need practice in making decisions, weighing options, and solving problems. Even children with limited cognitive abilities can practice making choices such as which shirt to wear or what snack to eat.

One simple strategy is to "think out loud" when we face our own challenges. Instead of quietly fixing a flat tire or rescheduling a conflicting appointment, we narrate our thought process.

"Okay, we've got a problem. The bus is running late, and we still must be at the doctor by 2:00. What are our choices? We could call a rideshare, reschedule the appointment, or see if Mom can drive us. What do you think is the best option?"

As we do this, we're modeling how to break big problems into smaller ones, how to consider consequences, and how to choose a course of action. When appropriate, we invite our son or daughter to make the final call. Over time, we also teach them how to speak up for what they need—whether that's asking a teacher for accommodations, clarifying instructions at work, or telling a doctor when something doesn't feel right.

Self-advocacy can be especially challenging for kids who've spent years in systems where decisions are made *about* them rather than *with* them. As dads, we can help shift that pattern by regularly asking questions like "What do you want?" "How do you feel about this?" and "What would you like to try?"

Discovering Interests, Passions, and Purpose

Independence isn't just about functioning; it's about *flourishing*. Our children are more than a collection of needs or diagnoses. They have interests, talents, and passions waiting to be discovered.

One of the best ways to foster independence is to give kids lots of exposure to different experiences: adaptive sports, Special Olympics, music, art, drama, cooking, STEM clubs, faith communities, youth groups, or hobby-based meetups. These environments do more than keep kids busy. They help them answer crucial questions:

What do I enjoy?

What am I good at?

Where do I feel like I belong?

Volunteering can be another powerful path. Helping at an animal shelter, participating in a community garden, assembling care packages, assisting at church or school events, all of these activities build a sense of usefulness and contribution. Our kids begin to see themselves not just as recipients of help but as givers, as people who make a difference.

I've watched again and again as parents describe a transformation. A son who once seemed uninterested in anything lights up around animals. A daughter who struggles academically thrives in a theater group. A young man who is quiet at home becomes a leader in a community project. Those sparks of joy and competence are clues. They point toward future possibilities, including employment.

Stories of Purpose and Employment

Some of the most inspiring examples of independence and self-sufficiency I've encountered have come from guests on the *SFN Dad To Dad Podcast*—men and women who illustrate what's possible when families, communities, and employers believe in people with disabilities.

One of the podcast guests was **Temple Grandin** of Fort Collins, Colorado, an outspoken advocate for individuals with autism and a renowned animal scientist. Temple's life is a testament to the power of understanding how a person thinks and learns, then building on their strengths. Early on, some professionals wrote her off. But her mother, teachers, and mentors gave her opportunities to work, design, and solve real-world problems. Temple has often said that young people on the spectrum need to be taught to *do things*—real tasks, real responsibilities, real work. She is adamant about the importance of employment, not just as a paycheck but as a path to dignity and purpose.

> *My name is Temple Grandin. I'm not like other people. I think in pictures, and I connect them.*
>
> *But here's the problem: Verbal thinkers get locked into labels. You're putting Elon Musk in the same category as an adult who is nonverbal and can't dress themselves—and you're giving them the same label?*
>
> *That doesn't make very much sense.*
>
> —Temple Grandin, *Dad To Dad Podcast*, episode #236

Another guest was **Mark X. Cronin** of Long Island, New York, who cofounded John's Crazy Socks with his son, John, who has Down syndrome. What began as John's love of colorful socks became a thriving business employing about three dozen people, roughly two-thirds of whom have disabilities. Mark and John's story demonstrates how leaning into a person's enthusiasm and creativity can lead to meaningful, sustainable work. Their company model shouts a simple message: *Disability is not inability; everyone has something to contribute.*

> **John:** *Hi, my name is John Cronin from John's Crazy Socks. My catchphrase is socks, socks, and more socks.*
>
> **Mark:** *You know, John is always looking to see what can we do for others. It's a simple idea. The more you do for others, the better off we are.*
>
> —Mark X. Cronin and John Cronin, *Dad To Dad Podcast*, episode #17

Another interesting guest was **Jim Stovall** of Tulsa, Oklahoma. An accomplished athlete in his youth, Jim lost his vision by age 29. His first book, *You Don't Have to Be Blind to See* (which I read thirty-plus years ago) was just the beginning; he has since written more than sixty books, eight of which have become major motion pictures, including *The Ultimate Gift*. Jim also founded the Narrative Television Network, making movies accessible to the more than thirteen million blind and visually impaired viewers. His life did not become smaller after vision loss; it became deeper and more impactful. Work, for Jim, became a powerful way to serve others and reclaim his own agency. He's also an amazing speaker, and I'm privileged to call him a friend.

> *I was exceedingly pleased when the movie* The Ultimate Gift *took off and became a sensation around the world. And that movie, and the two sequels and the books, have grossed over $100 million. [James Gardner's] share of that was certainly a whole lot more than we would have ever paid him. I think he may have made more money making our movie than anything he ever did. Sometimes, we don't get what we want, but as . . . the Rolling Stones said, we get what we need. It was what I needed.*
>
> —Jim Stovall, *Dad To Dad Podcast*, episode #163

Another insightful interview was with **Ben Mattlin** of Los Angeles, California, who was born with spinal muscular atrophy (SMA) and has been a wheelchair user his entire life. Ben is a nationally recognized disability rights advocate, a husband and father, and the author of several books, including *Miracle Boy Grows Up* and *Disability Pride*. His writing and advocacy challenge stereotypes and celebrate the disability community.

> *I've said this to newly disabled people—not to stigmatize it, and not to feel ashamed.*
>
> *When you learn about the disability community—what it's always done, how disabled people have always contributed to the world, to society, to culture—you can't help but feel proud. You can't be ashamed.*
>
> —Ben Mattlin, *Dad To Dad Podcast*, episode #258

Closer to my hometown of Chicago is my friend **Jim Mullen**, a Chicago police officer who was shot and catastrophically injured in the line of duty in 1996 and became a ventilator-dependent quadriplegic. His daughter, Maggie, was just 7 months old at that time. Most people would have understood if Jim had withdrawn from public life. Instead, he founded Mullen's food company, whose products are sold by major retailers (like Amazon, Costco, and Walmart), with proceeds supporting the Chicago Police Memorial Foundation and other charities. Jim still needs round-the-clock care, but that hasn't stopped him from building a business, giving back, and even enjoying the occasional ride in one of his vintage convertible muscle cars.

> *You do the best you can. We're all dealt a certain hand, and this happens to be the hand I'm playing right now. And you have to make the best of it, and do the best you can for your family.*
>
> —Jim Mullen, *Dad To Dad Podcast*, episode #215

Each of these stories is unique, but they all share a common thread: **With support, creativity, and opportunity, many people with disabilities find purpose in their productivity and contributions to our society.**

Preparing for the World of Work

Not every child will become a business founder, best-selling author, or public figure. That's okay. The goal is not fame; it's *fit*—helping our sons or daughters find a role that matches their abilities, interests, and support needs.

Preparation for employment often starts with small steps, such as showing up on time, following directions, communicating respectfully, accepting feedback, managing frustration, and staying on task. These "soft skills" are as important as any technical skill. We can practice them at home through chores, family projects, and community involvement.

As our children get older, job shadowing, internships, or volunteer roles can provide a first taste of the workplace. Supported employment programs, often run through schools, nonprofits, or government agencies, can help match individuals with jobs and provide job coaches who stay on site to teach and reinforce skills.

In episode #2 we featured **Randy Lewis**, the former executive vice president of Walgreens, who put it this way: "Successful businesses have to have a diverse workforce that reflects the community." Randy was a key leader behind Walgreens' initiative to build a distribution center in Anderson, South Carolina, and hire two hundred people with disabilities (out of the six hundred hired), proving that inclusive hiring isn't charity—it's good business. When companies take this approach, our children's opportunities expand dramatically. Dozens of companies, including Google, Microsoft, SAP, and Walmart, have made consequential commitments to hire those with disabilities.

> *From the get-go, we had to remember we're a business, not a charity. So if we were going to make this work, we said same performance standard, same pay, same jobs side by side. And I think that's what made it successful. If we were going to be able to sustain it, that was a standard we had to do.*
>
> —Randy Lewis, *Dad To Dad Podcast*, **episode #2**

As dads, we can advocate with educators, vocational counselors, and employers. We can ask about transition plans in IEP meetings, explore local supported employment services, and introduce our networks to the idea of inclusive hiring. Sometimes a single conversation or introduction opens a door that changes the trajectory of a young person's life.

Life Skills for Adulthood

Independence and self-sufficiency also involve the everyday skills of adult life. Over time, and at a pace and at a level that fits each child, we can work on:

- managing personal hygiene and grooming
- using calendars, alarms, or visual schedules to organize time
- understanding basic money concepts, such as earning, saving, spending, and budgeting
- learning to use public transportation, rideshare services, or mobility aids safely
- practicing communication, whether verbal, written, or through assistive technology
- recognizing health needs, taking medications as directed, and speaking up at medical appointments
- caring for living spaces—cooking simple meals, cleaning, doing laundry, and organizing belongings

We don't need to teach all of this at once, and we certainly don't need to do it alone. Schools, therapists, transition programs, and community organizations can help. But the message our children hear from us is crucial: *I believe you can learn. I believe you can grow. I believe your life has purpose.*

Family and Community: A Team Sport

Fostering independence is not a solo act. The whole family can play a part. Siblings can be allies and encouragers, not just helpers. Grandparents and extended family can celebrate progress and treat our children as capable participants in family life rather than fragile ornaments to be protected at all costs.

Community resources also matter. Adaptive recreation programs, faith communities, disability organizations, mentoring groups, and peer networks all expand our kids' worlds. They meet people who "get it," see role models further down the road, and practice social skills in real environments.

As fathers, our willingness to ask for help and to connect with others who share this journey is one of our greatest strengths. When we surround our families with a supportive network, independence becomes less scary because none of us is facing it alone.

Conclusion: A Lifelong Journey of Learning

Independence and self-sufficiency are not destinations; they are ongoing processes. Our children will continue to learn, adapt, and grow throughout their lives, and so will we. There will be setbacks, detours, and seasons where progress seems slow. There will also be breakthroughs, surprises, and moments of joy that make all the effort worthwhile.

As Temple Grandin often says, *"People need to be encouraged to think for themselves."* That encouragement starts at home, with fathers who allow their children to try, to think, to decide, and sometimes to fail. Mark X. Cronin reminds us that *"Everybody has a talent, and that talent has to be identified and nurtured."* Our job is not to script our children's futures but to help them uncover their gifts and put those gifts to work in the world.

When we foster a sense of independence and self-sufficiency—when we help our children build confidence, find purpose, and, where possible, engage in meaningful employment—we are doing far more than teaching skills. We are saying to them, your life matters. And that might be the most powerful message a father can send.

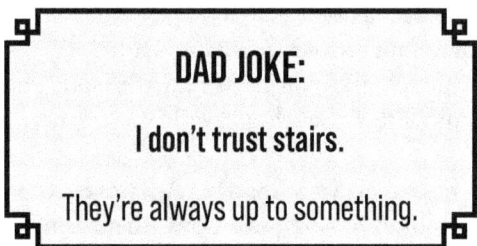

- 16 -
Protecting Your Family: The Importance of Estate and Financial Planning

RISE & SHINE

My child, you soar, no chains, no wall,
Strength within will stand tall.
Work is more than just a task,
It's purpose, pride—no need to ask.

Step by step, the world will see,
Independence lives in thee.

Disclaimer: The information contained within this section is not to be construed as specific advice to your circumstances. Always consult a competent attorney or investment professional who is licensed in your state (or geographic location) for specific and tailored advice. The ideas presented here are intended to provide you with a framework and some insights on important topics to consider for protecting your family from a legal and financial perspective.

When a child is diagnosed with a disability, everything in a family's life gets redefined: hopes, routines, expectations, even the language we use to describe the future. One of the most important shifts is financial. For many dads, it's the first time we realize that "providing" isn't just about next month's mortgage payment or next year's tuition. It's about decades—often an entire lifetime—of support, security, and dignity for a son or daughter who may never live fully independently.

That realization can be overwhelming. I've had countless conversations with fathers who quietly ask some version of the same question: *"What happens to my child when I'm gone?"*

Behind that question is a mix of love, fear, guilt, and a sense of responsibility. As a professional investment advisor for more than four decades, and as a father and grandfather myself, I've learned that the most loving, hopeful answer to that question is found in careful, intentional planning—especially special needs financial and estate planning.

This chapter is not about fancy strategies or legal jargon. It's about peace of mind. It's about preserving your child's public benefits, such as Medicaid and waiver supports, while improving their quality of life. It's about avoiding common pitfalls that can inadvertently harm the very child you're trying to protect. And it's about using tools, such as special needs trusts and working with experts—like some of the SFN Mentor Fathers I'll mention—to create a roadmap for your family's future.

When Disability Changes the Planning Equation

For families without a disability, traditional financial and estate planning can be relatively straightforward. Create a will, protect your family with life insurance, build assets, reduce debt, set aside funds for educational expenses, save for retirement, then leave what's left to your spouse and children outright.

For families touched by disability, that approach also requires parents to create a will, protect your family with life insurance, build assets, reduce debt, and plan for retirement but will include other factors as well. One of the great unknowns is "Will my child be able to attend college?" Also, what additional expenses will parents and caregivers need to address beyond the typical costs associated with childrearing?

One rule of thumb in the investment world is that for each child, you need to budget between $250,000 and $300,000 to cover four years of college expenses. For our family that meant $1,250,000, which fortunately we were able to do. This allowed our five children to graduate from college without any student debt. If your child is not likely to attend college, the funds that would otherwise be saved and directed to college can be used to meet more immediate needs and to fund accounts or trusts to support your child or children with disabilities.

In reality, many children with disabilities will rely on means-tested government benefits like Supplemental Security Income (SSI) and Medicaid for income support, health coverage, therapies, residential services, and long-term supports. These programs have strict asset and income limits. Leaving money to a child with a disability outright—through a will, life insurance, or beneficiary designation—can accidentally disqualify them from the very benefits that make their life sustainable.

I've seen situations where a well-meaning grandparent leaves a direct inheritance to a vulnerable grandchild, only to trigger a loss of benefits or bar eligibility completely until those funds are spent down. The money becomes a temporary bandage rather than a lifelong support. The intention was love; the outcome was instability.

Financial and estate planning for special needs isn't about "having more"—it's about structuring what you do have in a way that works *for* your child instead of against them.

Special Needs Trusts: The Cornerstone

That's where special needs trusts (SNTs) come in. If there is a single tool that every father of a child with a disability should at least know about, it's this one.

An SNT is a legal arrangement designed to hold assets for the benefit of a person with a disability without disqualifying them from means-tested government benefits. Properly drafted and managed, the trust can supplement what public programs provide—paying for things like education, transportation, therapies, recreation, technology, and experiences that enrich your child's life—while leaving eligibility for SSI and Medicaid intact.

There are different types of special needs trusts (often called "third-party" and "first-party" or "self-settled" trusts), each with its own rules and purposes. A third-party special needs trust is typically created by parents or grandparents and funded with their assets—through lifetime gifts or at death via their estate plan or life insurance. A first-party trust is funded with the child's own assets (perhaps from an accident settlement or inheritance received in the past) and has different payback rules. The details matter—and this is where specialized attorneys earn their keep—but the core idea is simple: **You want assets for your child to be owned and managed in a way that does not jeopardize their benefits.**

Setting up an SNT is not a DIY project. You absolutely want legal counsel that focuses on disability and public benefits law, because laws and regulations are complex, differ from state to state, and are constantly evolving. That's why I so deeply respect and lean on some of the expertise of SFN Mentor Fathers like **Brian Rubin** and **Rob Wrubel**, to name just two.

Brian Rubin: A Father, an Attorney, and a Guide

Brian Rubin is not just a special needs attorney; he's also the father of a son, Mitchell, now 45 years old, who has severe autism and other diagnosed special needs. His law practice—Rubin Law, based in Illinois—has, for decades, been dedicated exclusively to serving the legal and future-planning needs of families of children and adults with intellectual and developmental disabilities, mental illness, and related challenges.

Brian didn't just choose this niche as a business strategy; he grew into it through necessity and love. When Mitchell was born and later diagnosed, Brian realized that the legal profession wasn't built with families like his in mind. So he decided to change that. He became one of the country's leading voices on special needs estate and future planning, working day in and day out with moms and dads who are asking, like you, *"Will my child be okay when I'm not here?"*

In conversations, in publications, in podcast interviews, and at conferences, Brian has emphasized that planning is not merely about documents; it's about family dynamics. It's about thinking carefully about who will make decisions for your child when you can't, how siblings will be involved (and supported), how benefits will be preserved, and what structures need to be in place so your child can live with dignity and stability.

One of Brian's longtime areas of leadership is the Special Needs Alliance (SNA), a national, invitation-only organization of attorneys who focus their practices on disability, public benefits, and special needs estate planning. The SNA is a group of about two hundred estate planning attorneys who specialize in working with families touched by disability and (very importantly) have dedicated at least 50 percent of their practice to serving families whose loved ones have a disability. Rubin Law only works with families touched by disability.

While a local estate planning attorney may be willing, able, and well intentioned, I strongly recommend you start by finding an attorney who is part of the SNA (www.specialneedsalliance.org) and located in your area. Brian's life and work are a reminder that the legal side of planning is deeply personal. When you sit with an attorney who not only understands the law but also understands the emotional journey of raising a child with special needs, the process becomes less intimidating. You're not just filling in blanks on a form—you're crafting a future.

> You know, if somebody is higher functioning, maybe has Asperger's [autism spectrum disorder]. Okay. You know what? They can work. Maybe they have trouble working in a typical office setting. Never accept the fact that they can't do something. And keep that in mind when it comes to school, when it comes to employment. When it comes to living arrangements, it's: *I am going to look and see what's right for my kid.* Don't tell me these are only my three options.
>
> —Brian Rubin, *Dad To Dad Podcast,* episode #27

Rob Wrubel: Building Blocks for Financial Freedom

If special needs trusts are the legal cornerstone of planning, then financial planning is the structural framework that surrounds it.

Another talented SFN Mentor Father is Rob Wrubel. Rob is a financial planner, author, and father of a daughter with Down syndrome, based in Denver, Colorado. He has become a nationally recognized expert in financial planning for families with special needs members. His book *Financial Freedom for Special Needs Families: 9 Building Blocks to Preserve Benefits, Reduce Stress, and Create a Fulfilling Future* has guided many SFN fathers and others through the process of moving from fear and confusion to clarity and action.

What I appreciate about Rob's approach is that it's both practical and hopeful. He doesn't pretend the journey is easy, but he insists it is doable. He breaks planning down into manageable steps: understanding benefits, organizing finances, choosing appropriate insurance, coordinating with attorneys, funding special needs trusts, and revisiting plans as life changes. He reminds families that planning is not a one-time event; it's an ongoing process that evolves as your child grows, and as your own circumstances shift.

Rob's work underscores a critical truth: Legal planning and financial planning are two sides of the same coin. A beautifully drafted special needs trust that's never funded doesn't help your child. A solid investment or insurance strategy without proper legal structures can do more harm than good. The magic happens when the legal and financial pieces are coordinated thoughtfully.

> *In the special needs world, how are you planning for that kind of future? What does retirement look like? What is three years from now? So, a big part of the work you do and that I do is just giving people some space to dream a little bit and think a little bit. And then, we come back and put some structure around that for them.*
>
> —Rob Wrubel, *Dad To Dad Podcast*, episode #91

The Role of Organizations Like the Special Needs Alliance

No father should feel like he must become an amateur lawyer and financial planner overnight. The good news is that there are organizations designed to support you.

The Special Needs Alliance (www.specialneedsalliance.org), as mentioned earlier, is a national nonprofit association of attorneys dedicated specifically to disability and public benefits law, with deep experience in special needs estate and trust planning. Many of its members have family members with disabilities themselves, and the group serves as a kind of "seal of specialization" for families searching for qualified counsel.

Other helpful resources include:

- National and local chapters of the Arc and other disability organizations that offer future-planning guidance and referrals (https://thearc.org/our-initiatives/future-planning).
- The Academy of Special Needs Planners, which maintains a directory of attorneys and financial professionals focused on special needs planning (https://specialneedsanswers.com).

These resources exist so you don't have to figure this out alone. The hard work has already been done by organizations and professionals who live in this space every day. Your role, as a dad, is to take the first step.

Integrating Planning into Your Role as a Father

It's easy to think of financial and legal planning as something separate from fatherhood, as if love lives in one box, and paperwork, investments, and legal documents live in another. I see it differently.

From my perspective, sitting down to create a special needs trust, updating your will, buying appropriate life insurance, or meeting with a financial planner who understands disability issues is an act of fatherly love. It is another way of saying to your child, *"I see you. I acknowledge your needs. I am committed to your future—even beyond my own lifetime."*

Planning will require some difficult conversations. You may need to talk with your spouse or partner about what you each envision for your child's adulthood. You may need to bring siblings into the conversation and discuss what level of responsibility they are willing and able to assume. You may need to confront your own fears about mortality and about how much control you will or won't have over the future.

But something powerful happens in these conversations: Uncertainty begins to shrink, and clarity begins to grow. You start to see that while you cannot control everything, you can control *something*—and that something can make a profound difference.

Taking the First Step

If you haven't begun planning yet, or if your plan is out-of-date or incomplete, don't let shame or regret hold you back. Nearly every dad I know, including many of the most knowledgeable professionals I know, has had a moment of thinking, *"I should have done this sooner."* The important thing is not when you start, but that you start.

The first steps are to create a will and secure an adequate amount of life insurance to protect your family.

If you have a child, you need to create a will, one for you and one for your spouse or the mother of your child. In my four decades as a financial advisor, the one thing that seems to slow down the process of creating a will is *"If something happens to both of us, who will be the guardian(s) of my child or children?"* For some families, there is an obvious choice. For most, not so much so. The one piece of advice I can provide is that the guardian decision is *not* an irrevocable decision. Name the best person(s) based on your current situation and get your wills in place. The wills should be reviewed periodically and updated and changed as your situation evolves.

If you have a child, you need to secure life insurance. Remember, life insurance isn't for you, it's for your loved ones. Let me provide you with a simple framework for helping make this decision and offer my own biases. Figure out how much monthly income you'd like to provide for your loved ones. As an example, say you decide the amount is $5,000 per month or $60,000 per year, which I consider to be at the very low end. To generate $60,000 a year, assuming a 4 percent rate of return, you'll need to secure $1,500,000 in life insurance. In other words, if you're gone, and your spouse gets a check for $1,500,000, that money invested should be able to generate 4 percent a year or $60,000 a year without having to touch the principal. If you want to provide $10,000 a month, the amount of life insurance is simply twice that, or $3,000,000.

My Biases. For those who know me, and as mentioned above, I feel very strongly about securing an adequate amount of insurance. I also feel very strongly about not paying any more than necessary to secure that insurance. To keep it simple, there are three basic types of life insurance: whole life, universal or variable life, and term life. While there is a place for each of these, my bias is for term life, and more specifically, level-premium term, where your premiums are fixed or flat for either five, ten, fifteen, or twenty years. This is one of the most economical ways to secure the initial amount of life insurance to protect your family. This type of life insurance is supplemental to any coverage your employer might offer through a group term plan.

One more thought about life insurance. You need to make sure the beneficiary designations are done properly so as not to impact eligibility for SSI and Medicaid.

Please rely on someone you trust to assist with your wills and insurance. It might also be helpful to get a second opinion before you make your decision. Most importantly, be intentional and get these two building blocks of your plan in place as soon as possible. You'll feel good about making two important decisions, and you'll also receive some peace of mind for doing so.

Your next steps might be as simple as writing down your questions, gathering your existing documents, and visiting the website of the Special Needs Alliance to identify a qualified attorney in your state. It might mean ordering one of Rob Wrubel's books or listening to a podcast episode featuring experts like Brian Rubin or Rob Wrubel to orient yourself. It might mean blocking off an evening to talk with your spouse about what you both hope—and fear—for your child's future.

From there, you build: a trust, a coordinated set of beneficiary designations, a life insurance plan, an investment strategy, maybe an ABLE account, a written "letter of intent" that describes your child's routines and preferences, all supported by a team of professionals who understand your goals.

Piece by piece, choice by choice, you assemble a structure around your child that will remain even when you cannot.

Conclusion: A Legacy of Love, Not Just Paper

In the end, financial and estate planning for families touched by disability are not about documents sitting in a file cabinet or PDFs stored on a hard drive. It is about love translated into structure. It is about taking the deepest instincts you have as a father—to protect, to provide, to guide—and extending them into a future you will not see.

Special needs trusts, attorneys like Brian Rubin, planners like Rob Wrubel, organizations like the Special Needs Alliance, and the broader community of parents and professionals all exist to help you create that future. They are partners in your fatherhood journey.

The planning you do today will not erase every worry or eliminate every challenge. But it will give you something priceless: the knowledge that you have done what you can to secure a life of dignity, support, and possibility for your child.

And that, in my view, is one of the most important legacies a twenty-first century dad can leave.

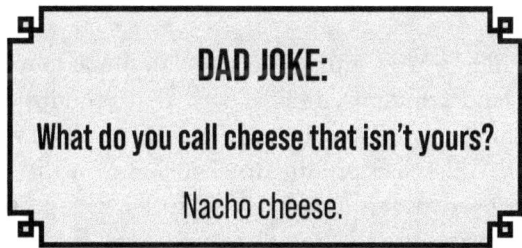

DAD JOKE:

What do you call cheese that isn't yours?

Nacho cheese.

- 17 -
Dads Raising Children with Autism: Navigating a Unique Path with Love and Patience

THE PATH IS YOURS

Through twists and turns, you find your way,
A world too loud, too bright some days.
But step by step, I walk with you,
Your mind unique, your heart so true.

No need to change, just rise and shine,
The path is yours—I'm by your side.

"Autism is not a disability, it's a different ability."
—Joe Mantegna

Disclaimer: This brief chapter provides a glimpse into some insights about autism. There is a growing body of research, including hundreds of books, thousands of research papers, and websites full of valuable information. See Appendix B for some additional resources.

Parenting children with autism presents a unique journey filled with challenges and triumphs. It is a path that requires love, patience, understanding, and an open heart to learn from those who experience autism firsthand. This chapter aims to shed light on the importance of learning from self-advocates, understanding their perspectives, and navigating the intricacies of autism with compassion. Through quotes from influential figures who advocate for individuals on the spectrum, we will explore how to best support and empower our children in their unique paths.

Understanding Autism

Autism spectrum disorder (ASD) is a developmental disorder that affects communication, behavior, and social interaction. The term "spectrum" reflects the wide range of symptoms and abilities among individuals with autism. Each person is unique, and understanding their specific needs, strengths, and challenges is crucial for fostering their growth and self-advocacy. The phrase often spoken within autism circles is *"If you've met one person with autism, you've met one person with autism."* What follows is based on research and informed by doing more than eighty interviews of those touched by autism.

Embracing Individuality

The individuality of children with autism means that there is no one-size-fits-all approach to parenting. Some children may excel in certain areas, such as math or art, while facing challenges in social interactions or sensory processing. As fathers, we must embrace and celebrate these differences.

Learning from Self-Advocates

Self-advocates are individuals with autism who speak out about their experiences, challenges, and successes. They offer invaluable insights that can help fathers understand their children better and provide the support they need. While doctors and therapists are well informed and highly educated, in most cases, they are providing professional advice. Self-advocates are speaking from their lived experiences.

Recognizing Unique Strengths. Self-advocates often emphasize their unique strengths and abilities. For instance, many individuals with autism possess exceptional attention to detail and deep focus in their areas of interest. As actor **Joe Mantegna** has stated, *"Autism is not a disability, it's a different ability."* This perspective encourages fathers to identify and nurture their children's passions, fostering self-esteem and confidence.

> *People say to me, "What's it like to have a daughter with autism?"*
>
> *I say, "I don't know what it's like not to." I can't explain that. Tough question. It is what it is.*
>
> *[Mia Mantegna from a video interview with her father, Joe]:*
>
> ***Joe:*** *What is your proudest achievement in dealing with autism?*

Mia: Today is certainly one of them. This one is right up there. The fact that I can sit here and be interviewed by you and be part of this Inclusion News interview—it's a very proud moment for me.

—Mia and Joe Mantegna, *Dad To Dad Podcast*, episode #5

Communicating Effectively. Effective communication is important in parenting children with autism. Self-advocates can provide guidance on how to approach conversations, understand nonverbal cues, and respect the individual's preferred communication styles. Listening to their experiences helps fathers develop strategies that enhance communication.

The Power of Patience

Patience is one of the most vital qualities a father can possess while navigating the complexities of raising a child with autism. Challenges may arise in various forms, from meltdowns to difficulties in understanding social cues. By cultivating patience, fathers can create a safe and supportive environment for their children to thrive.

Understanding Meltdowns. Meltdowns are common in children with autism, often resulting from overwhelming emotions, sensory overload, or an inability to communicate. Understanding the triggers and signs of a potential meltdown allows fathers to intervene early and provide the necessary support. Here are a handful of signals for identifying meltdowns and ways to avoid them:

- **Sensory Overload.** *Signs:* Covering ears, squinting or closing eyes, rocking back and forth, or verbal expressions like "It's too loud." *Avoidance Tip:* Minimize sensory stimuli. Offer a quiet, calm environment or noise-canceling headphones.
- **Escalating Anxiety or Distress.** *Signs:* Rapid breathing, pacing, clenching fists, or expressing frustration verbally or nonverbally. *Avoidance Tip:* Recognize triggers, modify the situation if possible, and provide reassurance. Use calm, soothing tones and predictable routines.
- **Difficulty Communicating.** *Signs:* increased difficulty expressing needs (among those who are able to communicate routinely), echolalia (repeating phrases), or complete silence. *Avoidance Tip:* Offer alternative communication methods like a visual aid, a notepad, or a communication app.

- **Intense Focus or Repetitive Behaviors.** *Signs:* Repeated motions, words, or fixations that become faster or more intense. *Avoidance Tip:* Respect the need for these behaviors but gently redirect when they become overwhelming or disruptive, or consider changing environments.
- **Physical Discomfort or Restlessness.** *Signs:* Fidgeting, scratching, hitting, or removing clothes to address sensory discomfort. *Avoidance Tip:* Ensure physical comfort by adjusting clothing, temperature, or seating arrangements. Also make sure there's no medical issue involved.

Here are a handful of ways to avoid meltdowns:

- **Understand Triggers:** Work with the individual to identify their specific triggers (e.g., bright lights, loud noises, sudden changes in routine) and proactively manage these factors.
- **Create a Safe Space:** Designate a quiet, low-stimulation area where the person can retreat if they feel overwhelmed.
- **Use Clear and Predictable Communication:** Provide visual schedules or written instructions. Warn about transitions or changes in advance.
- **Practice Sensory Management:** Provide sensory tools such as fidget toys, weighted blankets, or sensory-friendly clothing to reduce discomfort.
- **Stay Calm and Patient:** During escalating situations, try to remain composed. Offer validation for their feelings and allow them time to process emotions without added pressure.

Celebrating Small Wins

Each achievement, no matter how small, is a significant victory. Fathers should celebrate these moments, reinforcing positive behavior and motivating children to continue striving for success. *Tip:* Keep a journal of your child's progress and milestones. Reflecting on their growth can help you appreciate the journey and build a stronger bond.

Quotes from Influential Figures

Many celebrities and advocates have shared their insights on autism, highlighting the importance of acceptance, understanding, and support for individuals on the spectrum.

- **Tommy Hilfiger:** *"The world is a much more colorful place with people who have different perspectives."* Hilfiger's words remind us that diversity enriches our lives and that children with autism bring a unique viewpoint to the world. Hilfiger and his wife, Dee Oceleppo Hilfiger, have two autistic children.
- **Sylvester Stallone:** *"You have to keep your focus, and you have to keep your heart."* Stallone's advice speaks to the essence of parenting children with autism. Maintaining focus on your child's strengths while nurturing their emotional well-being is vital. Stallone and his first wife, Sasha Czack, had two boys, Sage and Seargeoh. Seargeoh is autistic.
- **Doug Flutie:** *"When you look at someone with autism, you see the challenges. But you also have to see the potential."* Flutie's words encourage fathers to look beyond the challenges and recognize the incredible potential within their children. Flutie and his wife, Laurie, have two children, a daughter, Alexa, and a son, Doug Flutie Jr., who has autism. The Fluties have been outspoken advocates through the Doug Flutie Jr. Foundation for Autism.
- **John Travolta:** *"I believe in the power of love and understanding."* Travolta's perspective emphasizes the importance of unconditional love and support in helping children with autism flourish. John and his late wife, Kelly Preston, had three children, Benjamin, Ella Bleu, and their oldest, Jett, who was autistic and very sadly died at age 16, in 2009.
- **Dan Marino:** *"The more you give to your children, the more they give back to you."* Marino highlights the reciprocal nature of parenting. The love and effort we invest in our children will often be reflected in their growth and happiness. Marino and his wife, Claire, are parents to six children including Michael, who is autistic. In 1992, shortly after Michael was diagnosed, they created the Dan Marino Foundation. The foundation has distributed more than $22 million to research, services, and treatment programs serving children with neurodevelopmental disabilities.
- **Eric Endlich:** *"Understanding autism is the key to supporting individuals with autism."* Endlich's insights underscore the importance of education and awareness in fostering an inclusive environment. Endlich and his wife, Kristina, are parents of two children, including an autistic son. Endlich discovered later in life he is also autistic. He is also the coauthor of the book *Older Autistic Adults: In Their Own Words, the Lost Generation*.

> *Autism isn't something you have any more than your race, gender, or sexuality is something you have—something you catch, get rid of, or that should be treated.*
>
> *It's just a part of who you are. I was born with a different brain. It works differently. So I'm autistic.*
>
> —Eric Endlich, *Dad To Dad Podcast*, **episode #213**

- **Sam Farmer:** *"The only limits are the ones you create for yourself."* Farmer's words remind fathers to encourage their children to break through barriers and pursue their passions without self-imposed limitations. Farmer and his wife are parents to an autistic teenage son. Like Endlich, Farmer was diagnosed later in life with autism. In addition to being a self-advocate, Farmer is also the author of the book *A Long Walk Down a Winding Road: Small Steps, Challenges and Triumphs Through an Autistic Lens*.

> *Realize there is a child behind the special need. There is a child in there who needs to be raised up and loved. They did not ask to come into this world, and we have a responsibility to raise them and give them the best possible shot—like you said, creating a longer runway for them. That perspective has inspired us to want to do more, not only for them, but for others as well.*
>
> —Sam Farmer, *Dad To Dad Podcast*, **episode #321**

Navigating the Unique Path of Fatherhood

Being a dad with a child with autism requires flexibility, empathy, and a willingness to adapt. Here are some strategies to help fathers navigate this unique path effectively:

Building Strong Relationships. Building a strong, trusting relationship with your child is essential. Engaging in activities that your child enjoys fosters connection and allows them to feel understood and supported. *Tip:* Spend one-on-one time with your child doing activities they love, whether it's playing video games, painting, or exploring nature.

Educating Yourself About Autism. Understanding autism is crucial for effective parenting. Take the time to educate yourself about the spectrum, common challenges, and strategies for support. *Tip:* Attend workshops, read books, and connect with professionals and other parents as well as self-advocates to gain insights and learn best practices.

Establishing Routines. Creating routines provides structure and predictability, which can be comforting for children with autism. Establishing daily routines helps children feel secure and reduces anxiety. *Tip:* Create visual schedules that outline daily activities, incorporating pictures and symbols to enhance understanding.

Collaborating with Professionals. Engaging with professionals, such as therapists, educators, and counselors, can provide additional support and resources for both you and your child. *Tip:* Establish open communication with your child's support team to discuss progress, challenges, and effective strategies.

Advocating for Your Child. Being an advocate for your child means standing up for their rights and ensuring they receive the support they need. This includes advocating for educational accommodations, therapy services, and social opportunities. *Tip:* Research your rights and available resources, and don't hesitate to speak up when necessary.

Encouraging Independence

As children with autism grow, encouraging independence becomes increasingly important. Fathers can play a pivotal role in helping their children develop the skills necessary for self-sufficiency.

Setting Goals Together. Work with your child to set achievable goals that promote independence in various areas, such as self-care, academics, and social interactions. *Tip:* Use the SMART (specific, measurable, achievable, relevant, time-bound) framework to create meaningful goals.

Promoting Life Skills. Teaching essential life skills is crucial for fostering independence. Focus on practical skills that will empower your child in their daily life. *Tip:* Involve your child in household chores and decision-making processes as much as possible to develop responsibility and confidence.

Encouraging Social Interaction. Social skills are vital for building relationships and navigating the world. Encourage your child to engage in social activities and practice communication skills. *Tip:* Arrange playdates or group activities that align with your child's interests to facilitate social interaction.

Finding Support and Community

Building a support network is important for fathers navigating the complexities of raising a child with autism. Connecting with other families and self-advocates can provide encouragement, guidance, and a sense of belonging.

Joining Support Groups. Consider joining support groups specifically for fathers of children with autism. These groups provide a safe space to share experiences, seek advice, and connect with others who understand your journey. *Tip:* Look for local organizations or online forums that offer resources and community support.

Engaging with and Learning from Self-Advocates. Listening to self-advocates can provide valuable insights into the challenges and strengths of individuals with autism. Engage with self-advocates through events, talks, or social media to learn from their experiences. (If possible, connect your child to self-advocates to provide role models and help foster disability identity development.) *Tip:* Attend events where self-advocates share their stories and perspectives, fostering understanding and connection. On June 22, 2024, 21st Century Dads Foundation hosted a Zoom panel discussion entitled Learning About Autism from Autistic Adults, featuring **Temple Grandin, Eric Endlich,** and **Sam Farmer,** which can be found on the 21st Century Dads YouTube Channel. Grandin, Endlich, and Farmer were also featured in separate episodes of the *SFN Dad To Dad Podcast.*

> Then she finally found Mick Jackson, the director, and Claire Danes. Christopher Munger, the writer, and they had the right team. And I think they did a really good job on the movie. But the producer was a mother of an autistic adult with severe autism, and she wanted it done right. And it shows my visual thinking exactly how I think visually. And it shows the sensory issues in autism. They did a great job with the movie. I'm very pleased with it. They shot all my projects and all the projects were in the movie I actually built.
>
> —Temple Grandin, *Dad To Dad Podcast*, episode #236

Celebrating Progress

As fathers, it's crucial to recognize and celebrate progress along the journey. Each milestone, no matter how small, is a testament to your child's growth and resilience.

Creating Celebration Rituals. Establish rituals for celebrating achievements, whether it's a special dinner, a small gift, or simply acknowledging the effort put into reaching a goal. *Tip:* Keep a "celebration jar" where you write down achievements and read them together during special occasions.

Reflecting on Growth. Regularly reflect on your child's progress and growth. Acknowledging their achievements helps build self-esteem and encourages them to continue striving for success. *Tip:* Create a scrapbook or digital album documenting milestones and positive moments, allowing you and your child to revisit cherished memories.

Conclusion: A Journey of Love and Growth

Raising a child with autism is a journey filled with unique challenges and profound rewards. It requires love, patience, and an unwavering commitment to understanding and supporting your child's individual needs.

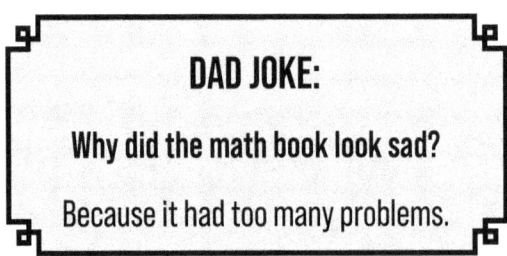

DAD JOKE:

Why did the math book look sad?

Because it had too many problems.

- 18 -
Supporting Children with Down Syndrome: Focusing on Abilities, Not Limitations

REDEFINING POSSIBLE

They set the limits, drew the line,
Said you'd be less, but you are mine.
And every day, you break the mold,
A spirit fierce, a heart so bold.

The world may measure worth in gold,
But love is worth more, truth be told.
For in your eyes, I see it plain—
A life of joy, not lived in vain.

Raising a child with Down syndrome is an extraordinary journey that opens doors to unique abilities and strengths. As fathers, our role is to focus on these abilities, embracing our children's potential while navigating the challenges that may arise. This chapter explores effective strategies for supporting children with Down syndrome, the importance of celebrating their achievements, and how to foster an environment where they can thrive.

Understanding Down Syndrome

Down syndrome, a genetic condition caused by the presence of an extra chromosome 21, results in a range of developmental delays and physical characteristics. However, it's essential to recognize that every individual with Down syndrome is unique, with their own personality, strengths, and capabilities.

The Importance of Focus. When discussing Down syndrome, it's easy for conversations to drift toward limitations rather than abilities. This chapter seeks to shift that narrative by highlighting the talents and potential within each child.

Focusing on Abilities. Children with Down syndrome often possess a variety of strengths, including:

- **Empathy:** Many individuals with Down syndrome are known for their warm, loving nature and ability to empathize with others.
- **Resilience:** Overcoming obstacles fosters a strong sense of determination and resilience.
- **Creativity:** Many children demonstrate exceptional creativity in arts, music, and problem-solving.
- **Social Skills:** Individuals with Down syndrome often thrive in social settings, forming strong bonds with peers and family.

By focusing on these strengths, we can empower our children to reach their full potential.

These SFN Mentor Fathers and influential figures in the Down syndrome community emphasize the importance of seeing the abilities in individuals rather than their limitations.

- **Nik Nikic:** *"Down syndrome is not a limit; it's a different ability."* As the father of Christopher, who made history in November 2020 at the Ironman Florida event as the first person in the world with Down syndrome to complete an Ironman distance triathlon, Nikic's words highlight the limitless potential of individuals with Down syndrome.

> *But if I can help my son to become the best he can be, maybe he can make a difference in someone else's life and then maybe that'll cascade, you know, around the world and make a difference for a lot of other people.*
>
> —**Nik Nikic,** *Dad To Dad Podcast,* **episode #108**

- **Paul Gianni:** *"The greatest gift we can give our children is the freedom to be themselves."* Gianni and his wife, Nancy, are friends and neighbors as well as cofounders of GiGi's Playhouse, named after their third child, Giuliana, who is also known as Gigi. The organization, with more than sixty locations in North America, including one in Mexico, supports individuals with Down syndrome and underscores the importance of acceptance and celebrating each child's uniqueness.

> *As soon as you have a child with special needs, it's amazing how your perspective changes.*
>
> *When you walk through the doors of GiGi's Playhouse, there's an overwhelming sense of acceptance and love. You just feel it—**we can do this**. It's a celebration. Lights are on. Smiles everywhere. Music playing.*
>
> *Today, there are more than thirty-three GiGi's Playhouses across the country. And it's not just about what GiGi's does for children and families—it's about what it does for communities. It helps build a better world, a world of tolerance and acceptance for the twenty-first century.*
>
> —**Paul Gianni**, *Dad To Dad Podcast*, **episode #6**

- **Lyle Liechty:** Cofounder of DADS (Dads Appreciating Down Syndrome). This national organization connects, supports, and empowers dads raising children with Down syndrome through shared experience, encouragement, and advocacy.

> *Don't ever give up. And be patient—because things will take longer. But they will accomplish things. . . .*
>
> *In general, I would say never give up. Because life is a marathon—it's not a sprint.*
>
> —**Lyle Liechty**, *Dad To Dad Podcast*, **episode #139**

- **Robert Hendershot:** The father of three boys, including oldest son, Trevor, who served as a greeter at Los Angeles Rams and Anaheim Ducks games, Hendershot saw how powerful employment was for his son. Trevor's experiences led Robert to create **Angels for Higher,** a national program to provide employment opportunities for dozens and dozens of young adults with Down syndrome.

> *He's worked ten years with the Angels, nine with the Ducks, and three with the Rams and the Trojans. Over time, he's become known, admired, and often loved by more than two million fans.*
>
> **—Robert Hendershot, *Dad To Dad Podcast*, episode #249**

- **Brady Murray:** He is the father to 11, including five adopted children. His biological son Nash and adopted son Cooper both have Down syndrome, which inspired Brady to create **RODS (Racing for Orphans with Down Syndrome) Heroes**, which raises funds to underwrite the cost of adoptions for children with disabilities. To date, they have funded well over one hundred adoptions, most of whom have been children with Down syndrome. Within RODS Heroes, there is a special program entitled Cooper's Mission. This program is an effort to unite thirty orphaned children with Down syndrome or other unique circumstances with their forever family—one pitch at a time, by raising funds in each community and making appearances at thirty Major League Baseball games.

There's a five-year gap between Ridge and Mason. Then we adopted Coop, and he fit right in the middle. It just felt like this was meant to be.

We learned about a little boy who had been abandoned on a street corner in a city of fourteen million people. He was believed to be about 6 months old. I can only guess it was because he had Down syndrome.

When we saw a picture of that little guy, we knew—he was our son.

—Brady Murray, *Dad To Dad Podcast*, episode #279

Supporting Your Child: Practical Strategies

As fathers, our support can significantly impact our children's growth and development. Here are some strategies to help you nurture your child's abilities:

Embrace Individuality. Every child is unique, and recognizing their individuality is crucial. Pay attention to your child's interests, strengths, and preferences. This allows you to tailor your support to their specific needs. *Tip:* Engage your child in conversations about their interests. Encourage them to explore various activities, from sports to arts, helping them discover their passions.

Set Realistic Goals. Goal setting is an effective way to promote growth and self-confidence. Establish achievable, specific goals for your child, focusing on both short-term and long-term aspirations. *Tip:* Use the SMART (specific, measurable, achievable, relevant, time-bound) framework to set goals. For example, if your child wants to learn to ride a bike, set a timeline for practice and gradually increase the challenge. Keep in mind the learning curve for those with Down syndrome is typically longer and will require a higher level of patience and perseverance.

Encourage Independence. Fostering independence is essential for personal growth. Encourage your child to take on age-appropriate responsibilities that promote self-sufficiency. Teach life skills step by step. *Tip:* Breaking tasks into smaller, manageable steps helps youth with Down syndrome learn and retain skills more effectively. Use visual aids, checklists, or videos to demonstrate processes like cooking, cleaning, or managing personal hygiene. Practice each step until they feel confident to proceed to the next. This not only builds confidence but also teaches important life skills.

Promote Social Interaction. Social skills are vital for developing friendships and navigating social situations. Social skills are also critical for independence in personal and professional relationships. Encourage your child to participate in group activities and playdates to build social connections. As mentioned previously, Special Olympics is one of the premiere organizations for individuals with Down syndrome to develop physically and socially. On the surface it's about athletic competition, but in reality it's about building community. *Tip:* Organize regular outings with peers or enroll your child in group classes where they can interact with others. You can also role-play scenarios to prepare them for real-life interactions.

Advocate for Your Child. As a father, being an advocate for your child is crucial. This means ensuring they receive the support and services necessary for their growth, whether in school or community settings. Here are a variety of ways fathers can advocate for their child with Down syndrome:

- **Educate Yourself:** Learn about Down syndrome and its associated health, developmental, and educational considerations. The more knowledgeable you are, the more effectively you can advocate for your child.
- **Partner with Professionals:** Build strong relationships with medical providers, therapists, and educators. Stay actively involved in your child's Individualized Education Program (IEP) or other support plans.
- **Engage in Early Intervention:** For parents of children 0–3, take advantage of early intervention services, such as speech therapy, physical therapy, and occupational therapy, to support your child's development.
- **Speak Up at School:** In addition to attending IEP meetings, work with teachers and administrators to ensure an inclusive and supportive educational environment. Advocate for accommodations, modifications, or services your child needs to thrive.
- **Raise Awareness:** Participate in local events or advocacy efforts to educate others about Down syndrome. Share your experiences to reduce stigma and promote understanding.
- **Build a Support Network:** Connect with other parents of children with Down syndrome through organizations like the National Down Syndrome Society (NDSS), Dads Appreciating Down Syndrome (DADS), or local support groups. Collaboration can amplify advocacy efforts.
- **Teach Self-Advocacy:** Help your child develop self-confidence and the skills to express their needs and preferences as they grow. Encourage independence whenever possible.
- **Get Involved Politically:** Advocate for policies and legislation that support individuals with Down syndrome and their families. This could include writing letters, meeting with elected officials and representatives, or joining advocacy campaigns.

- **Be a Role Model:** Demonstrate acceptance, patience, and resilience in your own actions. Your advocacy may inspire others in your community to follow suit.

Celebrate Achievements. Focus on your child's strengths and celebrate their milestones. Highlight their abilities to shift the narrative from disability to possibility. Finding ways to celebrate your child's achievements, no matter how small, reinforces positive behavior and encourages them to continue striving for success. Here are a variety of meaningful ways fathers can help their child with Down syndrome celebrate achievements:

- **Host a Celebration Party:** Organize a small gathering with family and friends to honor their achievements. It can be as simple as cake and balloons or as elaborate as a themed celebration.
- **Create a "Wall of Fame":** Dedicate a space in your home to display certificates, trophies, artwork, or pictures that highlight their accomplishments. This serves as a constant reminder of their progress.
- **Document and Share Their Successes:** Take photos or videos and share their milestones on social media or with your support network. Positive feedback from others can boost their confidence and sense of pride.
- **Celebrate with Their Favorite Activity:** Let them choose a fun activity or outing, like going to the zoo, having a picnic, or playing their favorite game, to mark their achievement in a way they enjoy.
- **Create a Personal Achievement Journal:** Work together to document their achievements in a journal with photos, drawings, or written notes. This can become a cherished keepsake over time.
- **Give a Meaningful Reward:** Offer a tangible token of recognition, such as a certificate you make together, a medal, or a small gift that aligns with their interests.
- **Involve Them in Sharing Their Story:** Encourage them to talk about their achievements with others. Whether through a family meeting or a podcast/video, this can empower them and build their communication skills.
- **Celebrate with Siblings and Peers:** Include siblings or friends in celebrating their achievements to help build strong social connections and foster mutual pride.

- **Acknowledge the Effort, Not Just the Outcome:** Highlight the hard work and persistence they've shown to achieve their goal. This reinforces the importance of trying their best.
- **Plan Future Goals Together:** Use their achievement as a steppingstone to set new goals. Discuss their aspirations and create a visual chart or plan to work toward the next milestone, showing you believe in their continued success.

Build a Supportive Environment. Creating an environment where your child feels supported and loved is crucial. Here are ways to foster such an environment:

- **Create a Nurturing Home:** A nurturing home environment promotes emotional well-being. Show your child love, patience, and understanding to help them feel secure. Practice active listening and open communication. Encourage your child to express their feelings and thoughts, validating their experiences.
- **Connect with Other Families:** Building connections with other families who have children with Down syndrome can provide invaluable support. Sharing experiences and resources helps fathers navigate the challenges of parenting together. Join local support groups or online communities to connect with other fathers. Attend events that focus on Down syndrome awareness and advocacy.
- **Engage with Professionals:** Incorporate professionals, such as therapists and educators, into your support network. Collaborating with them can enhance your child's development and help you learn effective strategies. Schedule regular meetings with your child's support team to discuss progress, challenges, and effective interventions.
- **The Role of Education.** Education plays a significant role in the development of children with Down syndrome. Advocating for inclusive educational practices can help your child thrive in school.
- **Encouraging Lifelong Learning.** Encourage a love of learning by providing diverse educational experiences. This can range from structured activities to informal learning opportunities. Incorporate educational games, field trips, and hands-on activities into your child's routine, making learning engaging and enjoyable.

Conclusion: The Power of Love and Acceptance

Supporting children with Down syndrome requires love, patience, and an unwavering belief in their abilities. By focusing on their strengths, celebrating achievements, and creating a nurturing environment, we empower our children to thrive and embrace their unique journey.

As we navigate the complexities of parenting children with Down syndrome, let us remember the words of Nancy Gianni: *"The greatest gift we can give our children is the freedom to be themselves."* This freedom allows our children to flourish, discover their passions, and contribute to the world in meaningful ways.

In the words of Nik Nikic, *"Down syndrome is not a limit; it's a different ability."* Let us embrace this perspective as we embark on this journey of love, growth, and endless possibilities. Through our support and encouragement, our children can achieve remarkable things and inspire others along the way.

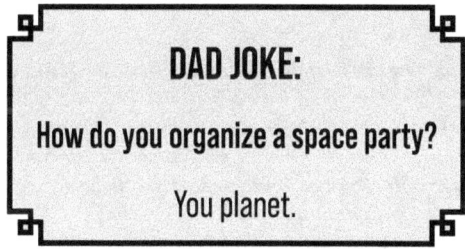

DAD JOKE:

How do you organize a space party?

You planet.

- 19 -
Rare Diseases and Resilience: Adapting to the Unknown with Courage

A FATHER'S HAND

These hands once built, these hands once made,
Now guide, protect, and softly braid.
They wipe your tears, they lift you high,
They push your chair when legs won't try.

But these hands know—they are not fate,
Not here to fix, nor to create.
Instead, they hold, they cheer, they show,
That love is more than what we know.

"Resilience is the ability to withstand adversity and bounce back from difficult life events."

—John Crowley

Disclaimer: By definition, rare diseases fall into two categories: diagnosed and yet to be diagnosed or undiagnosed. Among diagnosed rare diseases, there may be a single individual or as many as two hundred thousand individuals with the same condition. In most cases, the major pharmaceutical companies avoid research into rare diseases because the patient population is not large enough to provide an adequate return on investment (ROI) to justify the extraordinary investment required to identify treatments and cures. By some estimates, $5 million is the minimum amount required to pursue treatments and cures for a rare disease, a sum beyond the reach of all but a small percentage of parents and caregivers. The ideas included here are a primer for parents of a child with a rare disease.

Raising a child with a rare disease presents unique challenges and unexpected trials. These conditions, often defined as diseases affecting fewer than two hundred thousand individuals in the United States, can leave families grappling with uncertainty, anxiety, and fear. Yet within this struggle lies incredible resilience, the ability to adapt, grow, and find strength amid adversity. This chapter explores the world of rare diseases, highlighting specific conditions, their impact on families, and the remarkable resilience displayed by those affected.

Understanding Rare Diseases

Rare diseases encompass a vast array of health conditions that may be genetic, autoimmune, or infectious, often leading to debilitating symptoms or complications. Despite their rarity, hundreds of millions of individuals worldwide are affected by such conditions.

Even with the increased prevalence of genetic testing, the rare-disease journey has two main paths. The first is getting a definitive diagnosis, and the other is not. From the more than one hundred interviews I've done that include rare disease, most have received a formal diagnosis, but many others have not. So, the first step is getting the genetic testing done with the hope of getting a formal diagnosis, with the idea that knowledge leads to better understanding and a clearer path.

Here are some inspiring parents of children with rare diseases featured on the *SFN Dad To Dad Podcast*:

John Crowley: He is the father of three, including one diagnosed with Asperger's syndrome and two with Pompe disease, a lysosomal storage disorder. Upon learning of the Pompe diagnosis, John pivoted from his corporate career and became one of the most well-recognized advocates for rare disease, which led to a search to find a cure or treatment for Pompe, his leadership at Amicus Therapeutics, and now at Biotechnology Innovation Organization (BIO), the premier biotechnology advocacy organization representing biotech companies, industry leaders, and state biotech associations in the United States and more than thirty-five countries around the globe.

> *It's one of the great ironies of what we face with many special needs children—and certainly what we work on every day in the field of rare diseases. What we're really trying to give families is time: time with each other, time for those special moments, time to create more quality of life.*
>
> —**John Crowley,** *Dad To Dad Podcast,* **episode #71**

Hugh Hempel transitioned from a successful career in technology to full-time rare-disease research after his twin daughters were diagnosed with Niemann–Pick disease type C (NPC), an ultra-rare and fatal cholesterol disease that affects fewer than one thousand worldwide. Applying the same problem-solving, data-driven mindset he developed in tech, Hempel immersed himself in medical literature, built global research collaborations, and helped pioneer parent-led scientific efforts. His shift exemplifies how entrepreneurial skills—systems thinking, networking, and execution—can accelerate discovery and drive progress in rare-disease research when traditional pathways fall short.

> *The first challenge, of course, was finding a way to convince the FDA to allow us to treat our kids with this compound. We were fortunate to catch, as they say, lightning in a bottle, because it turns out this compound was being used as a delivery mechanism for another drug that Johnson & Johnson, through their subsidiary Janssen, had developed. Anyway, there was a drug master file for cyclodextrin that was created by Janssen. And we discovered that, and we asked them to help us, by sharing that drug master file, which they were reluctant to do. As you might expect, it was intellectual property owned by Janssen. And we politely asked them, and they refused. And then we not so politely told them that we thought that that was a bad idea.*
>
> —**Hugh Hempel,** *Dad To Dad Podcast,* **episode #412**

Ágúst Kristmanns: This father, from Reykjavík, Iceland, has three children, including his son, Ingi, who was diagnosed at age 11 with 2Q37 deletion syndrome, a rare chromosome condition affecting an estimated three hundred people in the world. Denied services for their son, the Kristmanns sued the education ministry. The controversy led to the creation of Einstök börn (which translates to Unique Children of Iceland), a nongovernmental organization (NGO) that brought meaningful change across the country for those impacted by rare disease.

> *We had to sue the ministry of schools and also the ministry in Reykjavík to get him into the special ed school classes. They constantly fought us with all their power.*
>
> *It took about two years of battling very, very hard on national news, in the papers, writing journal segments, and getting people to understand why we were battling it out. We got huge support from the special ed community and also from our community.*
>
> —Ágúst Kristmanns, *Dad To Dad Podcast*, episode #184

Allen Lynch: A Vietnam veteran, one of only eighty living recipients of the Medal of Honor, is the grandfather of Cailinn, who was diagnosed early in her life with a rare chromosomal disorder. In his own humble way, Lynch admits honestly that being a father and grandfather means more to him than receiving the Medal of Honor.

> *We did have to have hip surgery in January, where she was immobilized for six to seven weeks. The atrophy that happens when you literally can't move your lower body is astonishing.*
>
> *But she's walking—and dare I say it, she's running. She's chasing my dog around the house like she always has. And while there's a noticeable limp, she overcomes everything we put in front of her.*
>
> *She's a great kid. My wife and I were just remarking the other day about how happy she is. She's an extremely happy child—despite everything.*
>
> —Allen Lynch, *Dad To Dad Podcast*, episode #109

Swapna Sasidharan: She is the mother of two, including her 10-year-old son, Ved, who has POGZ, a rare genetic disorder characterized by developmental delays, cyclic vomiting, autism, microcephaly, and gastrointestinal issues. Motivated to find treatments and a cure, Sasidharan founded the Cure POGZ Disorder Foundation, with the goal of raising $5 million.

> *It did not bother my son that he could not walk any more than it bothers me that I cannot fly.*
>
> *He can be happy—so he chose happiness. And once you realize that, you stop worrying about whether your child will go to college, whether he will drive a car, whether he will get married.*
>
> *That realization gives you peace of mind and relief. And those things are what gave me strength.*
>
> —Swapna Sasidharan, *Dad To Dad Podcast*, episode #403

Are you a father of a child with a rare condition? Are you or the mother of the child on the fence about getting genetic testing done? Here are the primary pros and cons to help you make a more well-informed decision.

Pros of Genetic Testing for a Child with a Rare Disease

Accurate Diagnosis. Genetic testing often can identify the exact cause of a child's condition, leading to a more precise diagnosis that may not be possible through clinical evaluations alone.

Targeted Treatment Options. With a clear understanding of the genetic cause, doctors may be able to recommend more effective and personalized treatments, including experimental therapies or clinical trials.

Prognosis Clarity. Testing can provide insights into the likely progression of the disease, helping families plan for the future.

Access to Resources. A confirmed diagnosis often connects families to specialized support groups, financial resources, and advocacy organizations specific to the condition.

Family Planning Guidance. Results may inform parents about the likelihood of passing on the condition to future children, allowing them to make informed reproductive decisions.

Psychological Relief. Knowing the cause of a condition can reduce uncertainty and help families focus on managing the condition rather than seeking further diagnoses.

Advances in Research. Participating in genetic testing may contribute to broader scientific understanding, which could help other families in the future.

Insurance and Benefits Eligibility. A confirmed genetic diagnosis might be required to qualify for certain medical or educational services, therapies, or disability benefits.

Avoids Unnecessary Tests. Identifying the genetic cause can eliminate the need for repeated invasive or unnecessary diagnostic tests.

Siblings' Health. Testing may reveal if siblings are carriers or at risk, helping to monitor or manage their health proactively.

Cons of Genetic Testing for a Child with a Rare Disease

Emotional Impact. Receiving a genetic diagnosis can be emotionally overwhelming for families, potentially leading to feelings of guilt, grief, or anxiety.

Uncertainty of Results. Some genetic tests may yield inconclusive or uncertain results, leaving families without clear answers.

Ethical and Privacy Concerns. Storing and sharing genetic information raises privacy issues, and some families may worry about future misuse, such as genetic discrimination.

Cost. Genetic testing can be expensive, and not all tests or follow-up care are covered by insurance.

Impact on Family Dynamics. Results can affect family relationships, especially if other family members are found to be carriers or affected.

No Cure or Treatment. Even if a diagnosis is identified, there may be no available treatment or cure, leading to frustration or a sense of helplessness.

Stigmatization. A genetic diagnosis could lead to stigmatization or bias against the child in educational or social settings.

False Sense of Security. Negative results might lead families to underestimate the importance of continued monitoring or other health precautions.

Ethical Dilemmas. Testing could reveal unexpected information, such as nonpaternity or other genetic risks unrelated to the disease being tested.

Potential for Insurance Issues. While genetic discrimination is illegal in some contexts (e.g., health insurance via the Genetic Information Nondiscrimination Act in the United States), it may still occur in other areas, such as life or disability insurance.

With an estimated seven thousand or so rare diseases, it would be virtually impossible to cover all the bases. For purposes of providing you, the reader, with a sense for the nature of rare diseases, here is a list of more than thirty rare diseases, ranked by prevalence (most common to least common), along with a brief description of each. My apologies in advance if your child's diagnosis is not included here.

Most Common "Rare" Diseases

Sickle Cell Anemia. Prevalence: ~1 in 365 (African Americans). Genetic blood disorder causing abnormally shaped red blood cells, leading to anemia and pain.
Cystic Fibrosis. Prevalence: ~1 in 3,000 (Caucasians). Genetic disorder affecting the lungs and digestive system due to thick, sticky mucus buildup.
Duchenne Muscular Dystrophy (DMD). Prevalence: ~1 in 3,500–5,000 (males). Genetic muscle-wasting disease affecting strength and mobility.
Charcot-Marie-Tooth Disease. Prevalence: ~1 in 2,500–10,000. Hereditary condition affecting peripheral nerves, leading to muscle weakness and atrophy.
Marfan Syndrome. Prevalence: ~1 in 5,000. Connective tissue disorder affecting the heart, eyes, blood vessels, and skeleton.
Huntington's Disease. Prevalence: ~1 in 7,500. Genetic condition causing progressive brain degeneration, affecting movement, cognition, and behavior.
Spinal Muscular Atrophy (SMA). Prevalence: ~1 in 8,000–10,000. Genetic disorder leading to muscle weakness and atrophy due to loss of motor neurons.
Primary Biliary Cholangitis (PBC). Prevalence: ~1 in 10,000. Autoimmune liver disease causing bile duct damage and potentially leading to cirrhosis.
Amyotrophic Lateral Sclerosis (ALS). Prevalence: ~1 in 10,000. Neurodegenerative disease affecting motor neurons, leading to muscle weakness and paralysis. Although typically a disease affecting middle-aged adults, a rare form can strike very young children.

Moderately "Rare" Diseases

Rett Syndrome. Prevalence: ~1 in 10,000–15,000 (primarily affecting females). Neurodevelopmental disorder causing severe cognitive and physical disabilities.

Prader-Willi Syndrome. Prevalence: ~1 in 10,000–30,000. Genetic disorder affecting appetite, growth, metabolism, and cognitive development.

Angelman Syndrome. Prevalence: ~1 in 12,000–20,000. Neurodevelopmental disorder causing intellectual disability, speech impairment, and a happy demeanor.

Usher Syndrome. Prevalence: ~1 in 20,000–40,000. Genetic condition causing hearing loss and progressive vision loss.

Wilson Disease. Prevalence: ~1 in 30,000. Genetic disorder leading to copper accumulation in the liver, brain, and other organs.

Kabuki Syndrome. Prevalence: ~1 in 32,000–86,000. Rare genetic disorder characterized by distinctive facial features, developmental delays, and heart defects.

Von Hippel-Lindau Syndrome. Prevalence: ~1 in 36,000. Genetic condition causing tumors in multiple organs, including kidneys and eyes.

Pompe Disease. Prevalence: ~1 in 40,000–50,000. Glycogen storage disorder affecting muscles and heart.

Fabry Disease. Prevalence: ~1 in 40,000–60,000. Lysosomal storage disorder affecting multiple organs due to enzyme deficiency.

"Rare" and "Very Rare" Diseases

Alport Syndrome. Prevalence: ~1 in 50,000. Genetic condition causing kidney disease, hearing loss, and eye abnormalities.

Gaucher Disease. Prevalence: ~1 in 50,000. Genetic disorder causing fat accumulation in organs like the liver and spleen.

Sanfilippo Syndrome. Prevalence: ~1 in 70,000. Genetic metabolic disorder leading to neurological decline in children.

Ehlers-Danlos Syndrome (EDS). Prevalence: ~1 in 50,000–100,000. Connective tissue disorder leading to hypermobility, fragile skin, and joint instability.

Menkes Disease. Prevalence: ~1 in 100,000. Genetic disorder affecting copper levels, leading to developmental delays and weak muscle tone.

Niemann-Pick Disease. Prevalence: ~1 in 150,000. Lysosomal storage disorder affecting metabolism of lipids in cells.

Tay-Sachs Disease. Prevalence: ~1 in 300,000. Genetic condition causing progressive neurological decline.

"Extremely" Rare Diseases

Hyper IgM Syndrome. Prevalence: ~1 in 1 million. Immune deficiency causing increased susceptibility to infections.

Alstrom Syndrome. Prevalence: ~1 in 1 million. Rare genetic disorder affecting multiple organs, leading to vision loss, hearing loss, and heart disease.

Fibrodysplasia Ossificans Progressiva (FOP). Prevalence: ~1 in 2 million. Genetic condition causing connective tissue to turn into bone.

Progeria (Hutchinson-Gilford Progeria Syndrome). Prevalence: ~1 in 18 million–20 million. Rare disorder causing accelerated aging in children.

Kuru. Prevalence: Extremely rare, isolated cases. Fatal prion disease historically linked to cannibalistic practices.

Morgellons Disease. Prevalence: Unknown, potentially very rare. Controversial condition characterized by skin sensations and fiber-like material emerging from the skin.

Cloves Syndrome. Prevalence: ~200 reported cases worldwide. Overgrowth disorder causing vascular, skin, and tissue abnormalities.

RPI Deficiency. Prevalence: Fewer than 10 cases worldwide. Rare metabolic disorder affecting carbohydrate metabolism.

Fields Condition. Prevalence: 2 confirmed cases globally. Extremely rare neuromuscular disorder causing severe muscle degeneration and inability to speak.

The Emotional Toll of Rare Diseases

Raising a child with a rare disease often involves navigating a complex emotional landscape. Families frequently experience a range of feelings, including:

- **Fear and Anxiety:** The uncertainty of the condition, potential complications, and long-term outcomes can create fear and anxiety for parents and caregivers.
- **Isolation:** Many families feel isolated due to the rarity of their child's condition, making it challenging to find others who understand their experiences.
- **Grief and Loss:** The emotional burden can also manifest as grief, particularly when families mourn the life they had envisioned for their child.

Finding Strength in Adversity

Despite the emotional challenges, many families find remarkable resilience and strength. Here are some examples of how families adapt to the unknown:

- **Developing Support Networks:** Connecting with other families facing similar challenges creates a sense of community and shared understanding. These networks often provide emotional support, practical advice, and camaraderie.
- **Advocacy and Awareness:** Many families become advocates for their child's condition, raising awareness and pushing for research, funding, and policy changes. This activism can empower families and instill a sense of purpose.
- **Embracing Positivity:** Many families choose to focus on the positive aspects of their child's life. Celebrating small victories and milestones fosters a sense of joy and hope.
- **Seeking Professional Help:** Therapy and counseling can be invaluable resources for families navigating the emotional landscape of rare diseases. Professional support helps families develop coping strategies and resilience.

For-Profit and Nonprofit Organizations: Turning Loss into Hope

The emotional toll of rare diseases has spurred many families to engage in for-profit or to create nonprofit organizations in memory of their children or to support others facing similar challenges. Here are ten notable organizations associated with a rare disease:

Amicus Therapeutics was started to reimagine treatment for rare and orphan diseases and ultimately improve the lives of patients with devastating genetic conditions. John Crowley became CEO in 2005 and led the company through nearly two decades of growth.

Ainsley's Angels. *Cofounder:* Rooster Rossiter. Established to provide inclusive experiences for children with disabilities, Ainsley's Angels promotes inclusion in endurance events by providing adaptive racing chairs.

The Foundation for Angelman Syndrome Therapeutics (FAST). Founded by families affected by Angelman syndrome, FAST focuses on research and awareness to improve the lives of those with the condition.

The National Tay-Sachs and Allied Diseases Association (NTSAD). Established to support families affected by Tay-Sachs and related diseases, this organization funds research, offers resources, and raises awareness.

CureDuchenne. Founded by the parents of a boy with Duchenne muscular dystrophy, CureDuchenne funds research for treatments and advocates for patient access to therapies.

The Marfan Foundation. Established by individuals affected by Marfan syndrome, this foundation promotes awareness, education, and research for those living with the condition.

The Sturge-Weber Foundation. Created to support individuals and families affected by Sturge-Weber syndrome, this foundation provides education, resources, and advocacy for those impacted.

The Progeria Research Foundation. Founded by families affected by progeria, this organization focuses on funding research and raising awareness about the condition.

The Cystic Fibrosis Foundation. Established by families affected by cystic fibrosis, this organization funds research, provides resources, and advocates for improved care for individuals with CF.

The Resilience of Families

The stories of families affected by rare diseases demonstrate extraordinary resilience in the face of adversity. These families find strength in their love for their children, forming supportive networks, advocating for change, and celebrating achievements, both big and small.

Strategies for Building Resilience. Fostering resilience within families involves several key strategies:

- **Open Communication:** Encouraging open dialogue about feelings, fears, and challenges creates a supportive environment where family members can express themselves freely.
- **Cultivating a Positive Mindset:** Focusing on gratitude and the positives in life can help families cultivate resilience and navigate challenges with a hopeful outlook.
- **Embracing Flexibility:** Being adaptable and open to change helps families cope with the unpredictability of rare diseases.
- **Seeking Professional Support:** Accessing counseling and support groups can help families process their emotions and develop coping strategies.

- **Engaging in Self-Care:** Prioritizing self-care for parents and caregivers is crucial for maintaining overall well-being, allowing them to be more present and supportive for their children.

Conclusion: The Power of Resilience

Navigating the world of rare diseases requires incredible resilience and courage. Families learn to adapt to the unknown, find strength in community, and advocate for their children. As John Crowley eloquently states, *"Resilience is the ability to withstand adversity and bounce back from difficult life events."* This resilience not only empowers families but also creates a ripple effect, inspiring others facing similar challenges to embrace their journey with courage and determination.

Through their advocacy, support, and love, families affected by rare diseases shine a light on the beauty of resilience, transforming the challenges they face into a powerful testament of hope and strength. In a world filled with uncertainty, the stories of these families remind us that love and determination can conquer even the most formidable obstacles.

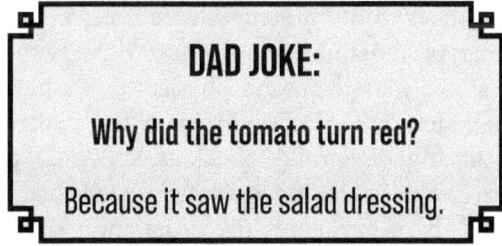

DAD JOKE:

Why did the tomato turn red?

Because it saw the salad dressing.

- 20 -
Cerebral Palsy and Strength: Overcoming Challenges with Determination

STEADY STEPS

Through each twist and turn, my child, you rise,
Strength in your heart, light in your eyes.
The world may not always see what I do,
But every step forward is a victory for you.

I'll walk beside you, steady and true,
Proud of the journey you're pushing through.

"Cerebral palsy is part of who I am, but it does not define me."
—Bonner Paddock, first person with cerebral palsy to summit Mount Kilimanjaro unassisted in 2008 and finish the Ironman World Championship in 2012

Cerebral palsy (CP) is a term that encompasses a group of neurological disorders affecting movement, muscle tone, and motor skills and results from atypical brain development or damage to the developing brain. It is one of the most common physical disabilities in childhood, affecting approximately 1 in 345 children in the United States alone. Symptoms can vary from very mild to serious. While CP presents unique challenges, it also provides countless stories of resilience, determination, and strength. This chapter explores the experiences of individuals with cerebral palsy, emphasizing their journeys, achievements, and unwavering spirit.

Understanding Cerebral Palsy

Cerebral palsy can manifest in various forms, often categorized into four main types based on the nature of the motor impairment.

Spastic Cerebral Palsy: Characterized by stiff and tight muscles, spastic CP affects voluntary movements, making it difficult to control limbs. It is the most common form of cerebral palsy.

Dyskinetic Cerebral Palsy: This type involves involuntary movements that may be slow or rapid, resulting in difficulty controlling body position and coordination.

Ataxic Cerebral Palsy: Individuals with ataxic CP experience challenges with balance and coordination, leading to unsteady movements.

Mixed Cerebral Palsy: Some individuals may exhibit characteristics of more than one type, known as mixed CP.

Despite the challenges associated with CP, many individuals have demonstrated remarkable determination and strength, overcoming obstacles to achieve their goals.

Stories of Strength: Voices from the Cerebral Palsy Community

The following are powerful quotes from individuals living with cerebral palsy, reflecting their experiences and the determination that drives them:

Geri Jewell of Orange County, California, the first person with a disability to have a regular role on a prime-time TV series, *The Facts of Life*. *"I'm not a disabled person; I'm a person with a disability. There's a difference."*

RJ Mitte of Los Angeles, California, an actor known for playing Walter White Jr. on *Breaking Bad*. *"Cerebral palsy is not a disability. It's an asset."*

Christy Brown of Parbrook, Somerset, England, who was an Irish writer and painter and author of *My Left Foot*, which was adapted into an Oscar-winning film. *"The only disability in life is a bad attitude."*

Dan Keplinger of Towson, Maryland, subject of the Oscar-winning documentary *King Gimp*; accomplished painter and speaker. *King Gimp* won the 2000 Academy Award for Best Documentary. The film also won a Peabody Award and was nominated for a national Emmy. *"Being different is just as good as being the same."*

Bonner Paddock of Laguna Beach, California, the first person with CP to summit Mount Kilimanjaro unassisted in 2008 and finish the Ironman World Championship in 2012. *"Cerebral palsy is part of who I am, but it does not define me."*

Still took a long time to kind of work through all of it. But at least in terms of the general direction, it made a snap 90-degree turn and was like, I'm going to spend the rest of my life trying to do something for all these other Jakeys in the world. So that I don't have to watch another family or experience that pain that I saw them have, because it was brutal to watch that and go to that funeral and everything else. So it really did springboard everything that I pretty much do now and my approach to life.

—**Bonner Paddock**, *Dad To Dad Podcast*, episode #230

Abbey Curran of Chicago, Illinois, the first woman with CP to compete in the Miss USA pageant, as Miss Iowa USA. She is also author of the book *The Courage to Compete* and founder and executive director of Miss You Can Do It, a national nonprofit whose mission is: *"Everybody has a disability; it's just that mine is visible."*

Maysoon Zayid, originally from Cliffside Park, New Jersey, a Muslim American comedian, actress, and disability advocate and cofounder of the New York Arab American Comedy Festival and Maysoon's Kids, a nonprofit dedicated to providing Palestinian children who have disabilities with the opportunity to be integrated into the mainstream school system. Her TEDx Talk has been viewed more than six million times (https://www.youtube.com/watch?v=buRLc2eWGPQ). *"If there's one thing you can do for a person with a disability, it's to hire us."*

Jerry Traylor of Phoenix, Arizona, marathon runner, motivational speaker, author of the book *Live CAREfully*, who climbed Pike's Peak in Colorado using crutches. *"I tell people that it's difficult to depend on others for personal growth. I needed to discover what I wanted to do on my own, and that allowed me to be the person I am. I always tell people that I'm not handicapped because I use crutches. I would be handicapped if I did not have crutches."*

Emma Livingstone of London, England, founder and chief executive officer of **UP—The Adult Cerebral Palsy Movement**, and mother of three typical kids. *"We're changing the way people think about Cerebral Palsy."*

If you have a child who isn't able to do those things, then we have a responsibility to provide opportunities where they can learn independent skills, learn to advocate for themselves, and have a voice.

—**Emma Livingstone**, *Dad To Dad Podcast*, episode #358

Overcoming Challenges with Determination

The individuals featured above highlight the resilience and determination of individuals with cerebral palsy. Their experiences illustrate the challenges they face and the strength they exhibit in overcoming them. Here are some common challenges faced by individuals with CP, along with strategies to foster determination and success.

Physical Challenges

Cerebral palsy often affects muscle control, coordination, and balance, leading to difficulties in mobility and physical activities. To overcome these physical challenges, consider:

- **Therapeutic Interventions:** Regular physical and occupational therapy can enhance strength, flexibility, and motor skills. Tailored programs help individuals build confidence in their abilities.
- **Assistive Technology:** Utilizing assistive devices, such as wheelchairs, walkers, or communication aids, enables individuals to navigate their environment and engage with others more easily.
- **Adaptive Sports:** Participating in adaptive sports provides individuals with opportunities to improve physical fitness, develop new skills, and foster a sense of community.

Social and Emotional Challenges

Living with a disability can sometimes lead to social isolation or feelings of inadequacy. To combat these emotional challenges:

- **Build Support Networks:** Connecting with others who understand your experiences creates a sense of belonging. Support groups, both online and in-person, can provide invaluable encouragement.
- **Self-Advocacy:** Encouraging individuals to speak up for their needs fosters independence and confidence. Learning to articulate their thoughts and feelings empowers them to advocate for themselves.
- **Mental Health Resources:** Accessing counseling and mental health support can help individuals navigate the emotional complexities associated with living with CP. Be sure to look for a therapist who is knowledgeable about disability issues.

Educational Challenges

Many individuals with cerebral palsy may encounter obstacles in educational settings. To address these challenges:

- **Individualized Education Plans (IEPs):** Working with educators to create tailored learning plans helps ensure that students receive the support they need to succeed academically.
- **Inclusive Classrooms:** Promoting inclusive educational environments fosters a sense of belonging and encourages peer relationships.
- **Assistive Learning Tools:** Utilizing technology and tools designed for learning can enhance educational experiences, making it easier for individuals with CP to engage with the curriculum.

The Role of Families and Support Systems

The journey of overcoming challenges is often supported by families, caregivers, and communities. Here are ways that families can foster strength and resilience in individuals with cerebral palsy:

- **Encouragement:** Offering words of affirmation and support instills confidence. Families should celebrate achievements, regardless of size, to reinforce a sense of accomplishment.
- **Involvement in Activities:** Encouraging participation in hobbies and interests helps individuals discover their passions and talents, fostering a sense of purpose.
- **Creating an Inclusive Environment:** Promoting an inclusive household, where individuals are encouraged to express themselves and engage in decision-making, nurtures independence.
- **Advocacy:** Families can advocate for necessary resources, services, and accommodations, ensuring that individuals with CP have access to opportunities that enable growth and development.
- **Celebrating Achievements.** Finding ways to celebrate achievements is vital to fostering a sense of accomplishment and motivation.
- **Recognition of Efforts:** Acknowledging hard work, whether in therapy, academics, or personal goals, reinforces the value of effort and determination.

- **Family Celebrations:** Creating family traditions to commemorate achievements—like small parties or outings—helps reinforce the importance of success.
- **Sharing Stories:** Encouraging individuals to share their accomplishments with friends and family cultivates pride and confidence.

Conclusion: Strength Through Determination

Cerebral palsy presents unique challenges, but the stories of those living with CP demonstrate the incredible strength and resilience that can emerge from adversity. Individuals with cerebral palsy, like Bonner Paddock and the many others highlighted in this chapter, inspire us all to embrace our challenges, strive for our goals, and advocate for a more inclusive world.

As we celebrate their achievements, we recognize that the true power of strength lies not in the absence of obstacles, but in the determination to rise above them. Each story serves as a reminder that, with courage and support, individuals with cerebral palsy can not only overcome challenges but also thrive in their journeys toward independence and fulfillment. The resilience displayed by these individuals inspires hope and reminds us of the incredible potential that resides within each person, regardless of the hurdles they face.

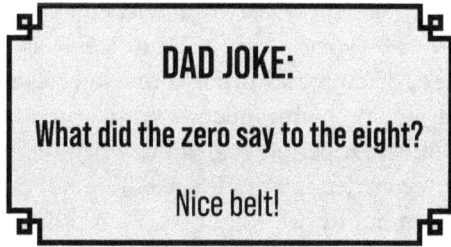

DAD JOKE:

What did the zero say to the eight?

Nice belt!

- 21 -
The Legacy of Fatherhood: Leaving a Lasting Impact on Your Family and Community

A FATHER'S IMPACT

I walk this path, my children in tow,
Guiding steps so they may grow.
Not just wealth, but love I leave,
A lasting impact of what I believe.

Legacy is one of those words we often associate with the end of a life—a summation, a eulogy, an inscription on a plaque or a name engraved in granite. Yet the longer I've lived, the more I've come to understand that legacy is not only something we leave behind; it is something we build every single day. It shows up in the stories our children tell, the memories they carry, the values they absorb, and the way they see their place in the world. Legacy begins in the quiet moments, the ordinary choices, the whispered encouragements, the late-night talks, the appointments we attend, the promises we keep, and the ones we wish we'd kept sooner.

My understanding of legacy has been shaped as much by what I did not receive as a boy as by what I have tried to create as a man. My father and I had a strained, distant, and often confusing relationship. As mentioned previously, I didn't see him much from the time I was 6 until I was 13, and there was a ten-year period as an adult when we didn't speak to one another. While we reconciled later in life, we were not close. Although we lived in the same community, we might see each other five or six times a year, mostly when he and my stepmom would attend one of my children's birthday parties.

Many of the good characteristics I inherited came from my maternal grandfather, Sam Solomon. We shared a loving relationship and a strong bond. He passed away when I was 40. He taught me about the importance of commitment to family, of living more frugally, and of serving others.

These lessons became the soil in which I grew, and like all early conditioning, they shaped the man I initially became without my realizing it.

After becoming a father, I developed the awareness to see how important those lessons would become. As the years passed and through the Illinois Fatherhood Initiative, I read thousands of essays entitled "What My Father Means to Me," written by school-aged children sharing what their fathers, stepfathers, grandfathers, and father figures mean to them. More recently, I've had the privilege of interviewing hundreds of men for the *SFN Dad To Dad Podcast*, about their own fatherhood journeys through the Special Fathers Network. I came to realize how common my story was. Many men were not running toward a model of fatherhood; they were running away from one.

Sometimes the most powerful legacy you can create is the one that breaks the cycle.

I didn't get to choose the father I had, but I did get to choose the father I would become. And that distinction—between inheritance and choice—has been one of the most important lessons of my life.

As a wealth advisor for more than forty-one years, I've spent countless hours helping families think about the future: their estates, investments, insurance, business succession, and financial security. These are important conversations, and I have always believed deeply in the importance of stewardship and planning. But over time, I've seen something that numbers alone can't capture. I've met families who amassed great financial wealth but struggled with emotional poverty. I've worked with children who inherited considerable estates, yet spoke about their fathers with more resentment than reverence. I've seen siblings fight over assets because they had never been taught how to talk about feelings, expectations, or fairness. And I've seen other families whose resources were modest but whose relationships were rich, healthy, and thriving.

I began to see that wealth can smooth the path, but it cannot fill the soul. Money can open doors, but it cannot repair the heart. A father may pass on all the tangible assets a child could ever need, but without love, time, honesty, presence, forgiveness, and connection, those assets lose meaning.

A father's deepest legacy is not financial—it is emotional.

And nowhere is that truth more vivid than in families raising children with special needs and disabilities.

When your child depends on you in ways other children might not—whether physically, medically, emotionally, or developmentally—the texture of fatherhood changes. You become not just a provider or protector, but an advocate, translator, navigator, and witness to challenges that most people never see. You learn patience you never thought you had. You measure milestones differently. You celebrate victories that others overlook. You grieve privately at times, worry silently, and yet find joy in places others might not recognize.

This kind of fatherhood deepens a man. It chisels him. It stretches him. It softens him. And it often reveals strengths he never knew were there. **Some of the best parenting I've witnessed is in families of those with special needs. Most of these parents, moms and dads, are more humble, less arrogant, and less selfish than the general population.**

Over the past decade, I've interviewed and worked with hundreds of men from all socioeconomic backgrounds, races, professions, and faiths, living in fourteen countries. Some were CEOs; others were truck drivers. Some were married; others were single or coparenting across complicated relationships. Some had children with physical disabilities, others with rare genetic disorders, others with emotional or behavioral challenges, and still others with diagnoses so complex that the medical field itself struggled for clarity.

And yet despite their differences, these fathers shared something profound: a fierce, unwavering commitment to being present for their children.

What struck me most was not their accomplishments or their strategies, but their stories—the late nights beside hospital beds, the endless paperwork, the moments of fear, the moments of awe, the breakthroughs, the setbacks, the conversations with teachers and therapists, the advocacy, the prayers, the laughter, the exhaustion, the pride, the determination. Their willingness to show up—again and again, even when it was hard—is the kind of legacy that endures.

I found myself learning as much from these dads as they did from the conversations we shared. Their resilience reminded me that legacy is not measured by ease but by effort, not by perfection but by perseverance.

Raising children with special needs has a way of stripping away the nonessentials. It forces you to become deeply intentional—not just about schedules and medical plans, but about how you show up emotionally. It teaches you to ask: What truly matters? What will my child remember? How will they describe our family someday? What will they say about me when I am no longer here to tell my own story?

These questions have become the compass by which I try to live. A couple of the benefits are that I rarely find myself having a pity party for myself or complaining about what people do, think, or say.

My journey into fatherhood advocacy was never part of a master plan. It emerged gradually—first through my involvement in the Illinois Fatherhood Initiative, then through the 21st Century Dads Foundation, and eventually through building the Special Fathers Network and hosting the *SFN Dad To Dad Podcast*. What began as a desire to learn how to be a better dad morphed into helping fathers engage more deeply with their children. About ten years ago, I realized it became a calling to elevate the role of fatherhood in our culture. Along the way, I discovered that being an outspoken advocate did not come from expertise alone—it came from vulnerability. It came from acknowledging my own wounds, my own shortcomings, my own longing for connection, and my deep conviction that fathers matter profoundly.

And fathers raising children with special needs matter in ways that society still does not fully recognize.

The commitment you make to your child—to understand them, support them, guide them, encourage them, fight for them, and believe in them—creates a legacy your child will carry for the rest of their life. It shapes their identity, their self-esteem, their sense of belonging. It influences how they treat others, how they assume responsibility, how they cope with adversity, how they advocate for themselves, and how they envision their own capabilities.

This legacy does not require perfection. It requires presence.

Being present is one of the greatest gifts a father can give. It is also one of the most overlooked. In a world driven by busyness, distraction, and constant noise, presence has become an endangered resource. Yet for a child with special needs, presence is everything. It provides stability, reassurance, and a framework for navigating the complexities of their daily lives. It tells them, *You matter. I'm with you. You are not alone.*

In my own family, I have come to understand that legacy is written in subtle ways. It's written in family dinners, road trips, bedtime routines, shared jokes, long hugs, hard conversations, and moments of forgiveness. It's written in apologies when I fall short. It's written in showing up at events even when I'm tired, or rearranging my calendar to attend a meeting that matters more to my child than any client ever could. It's written in the way I treat my spouse, in the tone I use at home, in the values I model, in the things I prioritize, and in the love I express.

I have also learned that legacy extends beyond the home. The way you engage with your community—the organizations you support, those you mentor, the time you volunteer, the men you encourage—these actions become threads in the larger tapestry of your life. As fathers, our influence is not confined to biological boundaries. Every dad who steps up inspires another dad to step up. Every father who learns becomes a father who teaches. Every man who shows compassion becomes a model for others. One committed father can shift the culture of an entire neighborhood, school, workplace, or congregation.

It's one of the most uplifting truths I've discovered in all my years of advocacy: Involved fathers inspire involvement in others.

Legacy is contagious.

Over time, I've also come to understand that legacy emerges not only from what we give but from what we choose to overcome. For many of us, that includes the wounds of our own childhoods. I spent years unconsciously wrestling with the emotional distance I experienced with my father. It wasn't until I faced it honestly—and chose to build something different for my own children—that I began to heal. Part of creating a legacy is recognizing what must not be passed down.

Breaking the cycle of father absence is itself an act of love.

This is particularly true for fathers raising children with disabilities. The path can be challenging emotionally, physically, financially, logistically. Yet every step you take toward understanding your child, every sacrifice you make, every advocacy effort you undertake, every moment of patience you summon, becomes part of the legacy they carry into adulthood.

Legacy does not guarantee ease. But it does guarantee meaning.

What has become most clear to me—through my work, my marriage, my fathering experience, and my advocacy—is that legacy is not a distant goal. It is a daily practice. It is woven through ordinary experiences, layered through consistent actions, and shaped through thousands of choices that may seem small in the moment but become monumental over time.

The question I return to again and again is simple: What will truly matter when everything else fades?

When I look back, I know it will not be the degrees I've earned, the achievements, or the size of my investment accounts. It will be the look in my children's eyes when they talk about their childhood. It will be the stories they tell their own children. It will be the way they treat others. It will be the values they carry. It will be the courage they have to navigate life with compassion and confidence. It will be the love they felt in our home.

That, more than anything else, is the legacy I hope to leave.

Reflecting on legacy and the Special Fathers Network, I see two paths: legacies not from raising a child, but from losing one, and legacies shaped not by tragedy, but by consistency, by how we choose to live every day.

Here are a few examples of legacies born from the loss and grief of losing a child.

When **Sam Rodriguez** lost his son, Manny, shortly after birth, his world shattered. The pain was permanent, but Sam and his wife, Stacey, made a choice that would redefine their lives. They would not allow their son's story to end with loss. Instead, they transformed their grief into service. They call it "87 Random Acts of Kindness." The 8/7 represents Manny's birth date, August 7. So, each year on Manny's birthday, the family goes out to perform 87 random acts of kindness. The Rodriguez family story teaches us that legacy does not require recovery from grief. It requires movement *through* it.

> *My heart was so full of love for him in that moment. They told us he likely had a genetic condition and wasn't going to live very long, and that we should take him off life support and simply love him and hold him. And so we did.*
>
> *From terrible tragedy comes forgiveness. A settlement was reached—an agreement—and we were able to take that money and put it back into the hospital. We even had the opportunity to sit with the doctors and tell them,* **we're not mad at you, we're not angry with you, we don't harbor ill will toward you.**
>
> *That choice led to incredible acts of kindness.*
>
> *Several years ago, my beautiful wife had an idea: Every year on his birthday—8/7, August 7th—we do* **87 random acts of kindness.**
>
> —Sam Rodriguez, *Dad To Dad Podcast*, episode #93

Harsha Rajasimha and his wife lost their middle daughter, Kahushi, to Edwards syndrome, a rare disease. They refused to let her short life be forgotten. Harsha went on to cofound **Jeeva Informatics**, a global rare-disease research collaboration, connecting families, scientists, and clinicians around the world. Kahushi's life became a catalyst for progress, innovation, and hope. Kahushi's legacy is a reminder that even the briefest life can leave a permanent imprint—and that a father's love can extend far beyond his own family.

> *Being part of a network of parents who are going through similar challenges makes a significant difference—for your child and for you. It helps you feel that you've done your very best to provide whatever support you could for your child.*
>
> —Harsha Rajasimha, *Dad To Dad Podcast*, episode #175

After losing his daughter, Lexi, at age 2, **Kris Kazian** created **Helping from Heaven: the Lexi Kazian Foundation**, a not-for-profit organization that improves the quality of life for families with special needs kids. He honored his child not through silence, but through action—by ensuring that other children and families would receive better care, better information, and better support. Lexi's legacy is living proof that remembrance can be active. A child's life can continue to shape the world through a father's courage to speak, lead, and persist.

> *I kind of fell into the fire service career—I've always believed in helping people. It's programmed into my DNA that you give back.*
>
> *Lexi was the most beautiful baby you could imagine, and we committed in that moment to take care of her.*
>
> *Sadly, Lexi passed away at age 2, about fourteen years ago. The fragility of life is something families raising children with special needs understand deeply—every day is a gift.*
>
> *Creating this nonprofit was my therapy after Lexi died. I love hearing her name spoken—it keeps her alive.*
>
> *Do everything you can to raise that child. Everyone has different means and abilities. You were chosen to be in that child's life—and you'll do everything you can, whatever that means.*
>
> —Kris Kazian, *Dad To Dad Podcast*, episode #31

Stephen "Doc" Hunsley, a former physician and father of three, lost his son, Mark, at age 5 to Dravet syndrome. Hunsley redirected his grief into creating **SOAR (Special Opportunities, Abilities, and Relationships) Special Needs**, which has become a steady presence for others, mentoring men, supporting families, and leading through example rather than spotlight. Mark's legacy is written in relationships, not recognition.

Hunsley reminds us that some legacies are deeply rooted, steady, and enduring.

> *People will say, "I don't want to talk about Mark—I don't want to bring up sadness for you." And I'm like,* **You don't have to remind me that Mark isn't here anymore. I wake up every day knowing that.**
>
> *But it brings me joy to talk about him and remember him. He's always going to be alive in my heart. He may not be here on earth, but he's alive in our family.*
>
> —Stephen "Doc" Hunsley, *Dad To Dad Podcast*, episode #122

These fathers teach us something essential:

Loss does not erase legacy.

Sometimes, legacy is born from it.

Here are a couple of examples of legacy born through the life we decide to lead.

After surviving a catastrophic childhood injury, **John O'Leary** could have lived a life defined by bitterness. Instead, he chose gratitude, optimism, and service. His legacy is not rooted in what happened to him, but in how he responded. John teaches us that legacy is often less about circumstance and more about character. The way a father lives after hardship may matter more than the hardship itself.

> *My eyes had been swollen shut, so I couldn't see. Because of damage to my lungs, I couldn't breathe or talk. I was a child dying in darkness.*
>
> *And into that darkness, I heard footsteps. I heard a chair scrape across the floor. Then I heard a voice—Jack Buck, the radio announcer for the St. Louis Cardinals—say,* **"Kid, wake up. You are going to live. Keep fighting."**
>
> *He said,* **"One day, John O'Leary Day at the ballpark will make it all worthwhile. Keep fighting."**
>
> —John O'Leary, *Dad To Dad Podcast*, episode #410

Larry Kaufman's legacy is defined by connection, generosity, and impact. A lifelong mentor, he has helped thousands navigate careers, transitions, and purpose by showing that relationships—not résumés—change lives. Long before "personal branding" became a buzzword, Larry mastered the art of meaningful engagement on LinkedIn, using the platform to open doors, spark introductions, and create opportunity at scale. His book, *The NCG Factor: A Formula for Building Life-Changing Relationships from College to Retirement*, distills decades of wisdom into a practical, human-centered guide for building authentic networks. Larry's enduring gift is teaching people how to help others—and, in doing so, help themselves.

> *He saw me. I saw him. He came over and gave me a hug and said, "I'm sorry."*
>
> *I said, "What?"*
>
> *He said, "I was terrible to you in junior high, and I want to apologize for my behavior. I went to high school with the same guys who were bullying you, but I parted ways from them. I realized it was wrong. I'm glad I could see you and apologize and say I'm sorry."*
>
> —**Larry Kaufman**, *Dad To Dad Podcast*, episode #146

Conclusion: A Final Reflection on What Will Matter Most

After more than forty-one years helping families build their financial futures, after decades of raising my own children, after interviewing hundreds of extraordinary dads, and after dedicating much of my adult life to fatherhood advocacy, here is what I know with absolute certainty:

Your legacy is not what you leave *for* your children.
Your legacy is what you leave *in* your children.

Love. Courage. Compassion. Resilience. Belief. Belonging. Confidence. Identity. Service. Hope.

These are the gifts that last.
These are the gifts that echo across generations.
These are the gifts that shape communities.
These are the gifts that define your life as a father.

And the beautiful part of legacy is this: It is never too early to begin and never too late to change.

Legacy is not something you write at the end of your life. It is something you live every day.

And the world needs fathers who are willing to lead with love, purpose, and presence—especially fathers raising children with special needs and abilities.

This is the legacy I strive to leave.
It is the legacy I invite you to create.
And it is the legacy our children—and our communities—deserve.

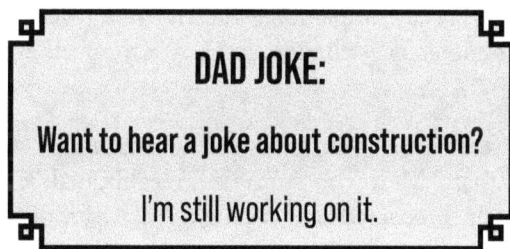

DAD JOKE:

Want to hear a joke about construction?

I'm still working on it.

Epilogue
The Journey Continues

To the fathers, stepfathers, grandfathers, father figures, and caregivers walking this road—welcome to the moment where reflection meets resolve.

If you have reached these final pages, you have already demonstrated something powerful: commitment. Not perfection. Not certainty. Commitment. The kind that shows up day after day, often quietly, often exhausted, often unseen. The kind that chooses presence over comfort and love over fear.

Dads Raising Children with Special Needs and Dis***abilities*** was never intended to be read once and shelved. It is not a checklist to complete or a manual to master. It is a companion—meant to be revisited as your child grows, as your circumstances change, and as you yourself evolve as a father and as a man.

Throughout these chapters, you have heard from fathers who have "been there and done that." Men who stumbled, recalibrated, learned the hard way, and ultimately discovered that raising a child with disabilities is not a detour from meaningful fatherhood—it is a deeper invitation into it. Their stories, alongside your own lived experience, form a shared understanding of what modern fatherhood truly looks like: adaptive, courageous, emotionally engaged, and grounded in dignity.

At its core, this book is about **seeing your child fully**—not through the lens of diagnosis or limitation, but through possibility, character, effort, and humanity. It is about learning when to advocate fiercely and when to step back with trust. When to protect, and when to let go just enough to allow growth. Independence, as you have read, is not about distance—it is about dignity.

That is why the curriculum included in the back of this book matters so deeply.

The curriculum is not supplemental—it is foundational. It is where insight becomes practice. Where reflection turns into action. Where big ideas are translated into small, repeatable steps that can be lived out in real kitchens, classrooms, doctor's offices, workplaces, and quiet moments with your child.

Use it intentionally.

Return to it when you feel overwhelmed.
Work through it when a new challenge emerges.
Share it with a partner, a support group, a therapist, a coach, or another dad who is just beginning this journey.

The prompts, exercises, and reflections are designed to help you slow down, ask better questions, and build confidence—both yours and your child's. They are meant to support conversations that matter, decisions that feel heavy, and moments that deserve celebration but often pass unnoticed.

And perhaps most importantly, they remind you that **you do not have to do this alone.**

There is a quiet myth that fathers are supposed to "figure it out," shoulder the weight, and push through. This book stands firmly against that myth. Strength is not isolation. Leadership is not silence. The strongest fathers are learners, listeners, and builders of community.

As you close this book, know this: The path ahead may still include uncertainty, frustration, advocacy battles, and moments of deep fatigue. But it will also be rich with connection, laughter, pride, unexpected joy, and love that reshapes you in ways you could not have imagined.

Your presence matters.
Your voice matters.
Your belief in your child matters.

The legacy you are creating is not measured by milestones alone, but by the safety, confidence, and worth your child feels because you showed up—again and again.

So take what you have learned here.
Return to it often.
Live it imperfectly and wholeheartedly.

Life is, indeed, a journey.

Enjoy the ride—and know that the road you are on is meaningful, necessary, and filled with purpose.

Curriculum: A Resource for Further Reflection

How to Make the Best Use of This Curriculum

Purpose

This curriculum was created to support fathers raising children with special needs and abilities through meaningful conversation, reflection, and action. While the book itself offers stories, insights, and guidance, this curriculum is designed to **activate** the content—helping dads move from reading to reflecting, and ultimately to resolving how they will show up differently as fathers, partners, advocates, and men.

This curriculum is intentionally simple, flexible, and respectful of the realities fathers face. It is not therapy. It is not a lecture series. It is a structured conversation tool that creates a safe space for honesty, learning, connection, and growth.

You will benefit greatly if you can meet with other fathers to discuss these questions, because when we listen, support, and hold one another accountable, we increase our opportunity for growth in our fathering. So, get together with some other dads, and see where this curriculum can take you. (While the sessions are designed to stimulate discussion in small groups, they can also be studied individually or with your spouse.)

Who This Curriculum Is For

This curriculum is designed for use by individual dads using the questions for personal reflection, small groups of dads (three to eight participants is ideal), mastermind groups and peer-support circles, faith-based, nonprofit, health-care, or community-based father groups.

The Read-Reflect-Resolve Framework

Each session uses a consistent three-part framework:

Read—Anchors the discussion in a core idea from the chapter. This ensures everyone is grounded in the same theme, even if participants are at different places in their fatherhood journey.

Reflect—Invites fathers to look inward. These questions are designed to encourage personal insight, emotional awareness, and connection to lived experience. Silence is allowed here. Reflection takes time.

Resolve—Moves the conversation from insight to action. These questions help fathers identify one small, practical step they can take. Progress, not perfection, is the goal.

A Note to Facilitators

No facilitation background is required. The most important qualification for a facilitator is the willingness to listen, respect confidentiality, and model authenticity.

As a facilitator, your role is not to force equal time or perfect answers, but to help the group move through these three stages intentionally.

Creating a Safe and Trustworthy Environment

Psychological safety is essential. Fathers will only share honestly if they believe the group is safe. It is strongly recommended to establish the following ground rules at the beginning of the first session:

1. **Confidentiality**–What is shared in the group stays in the group.
2. **No Fixing**–This is not a problem-solving competition. Listening is more important than advising.
3. **Respect Different Journeys**–Every child, diagnosis, family structure, and fatherhood path is different.
4. **Speak from Personal Experience**–Use "I" statements rather than generalizations.
5. **Silence Is Okay**–No one is required to share on every question.

Revisit these norms briefly at the start of each session, especially when new participants join.

Group Size and Session Length

Ideal group size: Three to eight dads
Recommended session length: 60–90 minutes

A typical session might look like this: Welcome and check-in: 5–10 minutes; Chapter discussion: 35–50 minutes; Resolve commitments and closing reflections: 10–15 minutes.

Groups may choose to cover one session at a time or, in longer meetings, two related chapters.

Facilitator Posture: Lead by Guiding, Not Teaching

Facilitators are not expected to be experts. In fact, groups are often strongest when facilitators model vulnerability rather than authority.

Helpful facilitation practices include:

- Asking open-ended follow-up questions ("Can you say more about that?")
- Reflecting back what you hear ("It sounds like that was a turning point for you")
- Normalizing emotions ("Many dads here have felt that way")
- Gently redirecting if one voice dominates

Avoid:

- Lecturing
- Comparing whose situation is harder (i.e., the "hardship Olympics")
- Offering unsolicited advice
- Rushing the conversation

Using the Questions Effectively

Each session includes five sections with questions about each. You do not need to cover all five every time.

Options include choosing a few questions based on group energy, letting the group vote on which questions resonate most, or spending an entire session on a single powerful question.

Depth matters more than coverage.

Handling Strong Emotions

Discussions may surface grief, anger, fear, guilt, or sadness. This is normal.

As a facilitator, acknowledge the emotion, thank the dad for his honesty, pause if needed, or offer a brief grounding moment (deep breath, silence).

You are not responsible for resolving these emotions—only for holding space.

If a participant appears overwhelmed, follow up privately after the session and, if appropriate, encourage professional support.

Accountability Without Pressure

The Resolve questions invite action, but they are not meant to create guilt or pressure.

Encourage participants to choose small, achievable steps, share only what they're comfortable committing to, and view setbacks as learning, not failure.

Some groups find it helpful to begin each session by briefly revisiting prior commitments, always with grace.

Adapting for Different Contexts

This curriculum is intentionally adaptable:

- **Mentor/Mentee pairs:** Use questions conversationally over multiple shorter meetings.
- **Virtual groups:** Encourage cameras on, mute notifications, and use breakout rooms if needed.
- **Faith-based groups:** Add optional prayer or reflection aligned with your tradition.
- **Individual use:** Journal responses and revisit Resolve commitments weekly.

Closing Each Session

Consider ending sessions with one of the following:

- A single-word checkout ("How are you leaving today?")
- A shared reflection sentence ("One thing I'm taking with me is...")
- The chapter's dad joke (humor matters)

Consistency in closing builds trust and rhythm.

Final Encouragement to Facilitators

Facilitating these conversations is an act of service. By creating a safe space for fathers to speak honestly—sometimes for the first time—you are strengthening families, modeling healthy masculinity, and helping break cycles of isolation.

You do not need to have all the answers. Your presence is enough.

Chapter 1 | Redefining Fatherhood: The Journey of Raising a Child with Special Abilities

1. The Story I Thought I Was Living

READ:

The chapter describes grieving the imagined future while discovering a new one.

REFLECT:

What did you *expect* fatherhood to look like before your child's diagnosis?

What parts of that vision have been hardest to release?

RESOLVE:

Identify one expectation you are willing to consciously let go of this month—and one new possibility you are willing to explore instead.

2. From "What's Wrong?" to "What's Strong?"

READ:

The chapter challenges fathers to focus on abilities rather than deficits.

REFLECT:

When you think about your child, what strengths or abilities come to mind first?

How often do those strengths get overshadowed by challenges, appointments, or comparisons?

RESOLVE:

Commit to noticing and naming one strength in your child every day this week—out loud, to them or to someone else.

3. Redefining What Success Looks Like

READ:

"Strength in small steps" reframes progress and milestones.

REFLECT:

What "small steps" has your child taken that others might overlook—but you know are huge?

How has your definition of success changed since becoming
a father to a child with special abilities?

RESOLVE:

Choose one recent small win and decide how you will celebrate
it—personally, as a family, or within your support circle.

4. The Father You Are Becoming

READ:

The chapter emphasizes how this journey reshapes *you* as a father and as a man.

REFLECT:

In what ways has this journey made you more patient, present, or resilient?

What qualities has your child drawn out of you that
might not have emerged otherwise?

RESOLVE:

Name one way you want to show up more intentionally
as a father in the next thirty days.

5. I Wouldn't Change a Thing

READ:

The chapter closes with a statement many dads eventually come to believe.

REFLECT:

How do you react to the phrase:
"Knowing everything I know today, I would not change a thing"?

Does it feel true, uncomfortable, hopeful—or all three?

RESOLVE:

Write (or share) one sentence completing this thought:

"This journey has taught me _____."

Optional Close:

Complete or have each dad complete this sentence:

"My family is strongest when we _____ together."

Chapter 2 | Strength Through Unity: The Power of Marriage in Navigating Special Needs

1. Unity Under Pressure

READ:

The chapter frames marriage or partnership as a *united front* rather than a perfect relationship.

REFLECT:

In what ways do you and your partner or coparent currently feel united?

Where does stress most often create distance or misunderstanding?

RESOLVE:

Identify one intentional action you can take this week to reinforce unity, however small.

2. The Weight We Carry

READ:

Special needs parenting magnifies emotional, physical, and mental strain.

REFLECT:

What part of this journey feels heaviest for you right now?

How openly is that weight shared with your partner or support system?

RESOLVE:

Commit to naming one burden out loud to your partner, a trusted friend, or a mentor.

3. Communication When It's Hardest

READ:

The chapter emphasizes honest, empathetic communication over problem-solving.

REFLECT:

When stress rises, do you tend to talk more, shut down, or try to fix things quickly?

How does your partner or coparent communicate differently?

RESOLVE:

Schedule one short, intentional check-in focused only on listening.

4. Teamwork vs. Scorekeeping

READ:

Strong partnerships focus on collaboration, not comparison.

REFLECT:

Where might scorekeeping—spoken or unspoken— be creeping into your relationship?

How could tasks or responsibilities be better aligned with each person's strengths?

RESOLVE:

Choose one responsibility to share, shift, or release with trust.

5. Protecting the Relationship

READ:

The chapter reminds us that the partnership must be nurtured as well as the child.

REFLECT:

How has your relationship changed since becoming a special needs parent?

What kind of connection do you want to rebuild or strengthen?

RESOLVE:

Plan one simple moment of connection this week— time, touch, gratitude, or humor.

Optional Close:

Complete or have each dad complete this sentence (spoken or written):

"**Our family is strongest when we remember that we're_____.**"

Chapter 3 | Grieving the Life You Anticipated: Finding Peace in the New Reality

1. Naming the Grief

READ:

Grief often comes from lost expectations, not lost love.

REFLECT:

What dreams or expectations have you quietly grieved?

How have you allowed—or avoided—those emotions?

RESOLVE:

Acknowledge one loss honestly, without minimizing it.

2. Grief and Identity

READ:

Fatherhood can reshape how we see ourselves.

REFLECT:

How has raising a child with special needs changed your identity as a man or father?

Where do you feel strongest—and where do you feel uncertain?

RESOLVE:

Offer yourself grace in one area where you feel inadequate.

3. Moving Toward Acceptance

READ:

Acceptance allows space for peace and growth.

REFLECT:

What does acceptance mean to you—right now, not someday?

Where are you still stuck in "should have" or "what if" thinking?

RESOLVE:

Practice staying present when those thoughts arise.

4. Finding Joy Again

READ:

Joy can coexist with grief.

REFLECT:

What moments with your child bring you genuine joy today?

How do you allow yourself to experience joy without guilt?

RESOLVE:

Intentionally create one joyful moment this week.

5. Building a New Vision

READ:

The future can still hold purpose and meaning.

REFLECT:

What does a fulfilling future look like now—for you and your family?

What values will guide that vision?

RESOLVE:

Write one sentence describing the future you're choosing to build.

Optional Close:

"Peace comes when I stop fighting reality and start living it."

Chapter 4 | Being Present: Physically, Emotionally, and Spiritually for Your Child

1. Presence Beyond Providing

READ:

The chapter challenges the idea that a father's primary role is financial provision.

REFLECT:

When you think about being a "good provider," what comes to mind first—money, time, or presence?

In what ways might your child need *you* more than what you provide?

RESOLVE:

Identify one way you can show up this week that has nothing to do with money.

2. Showing Up—and Staying Engaged

READ:

Physical presence is described as active participation, not just being nearby.

REFLECT:

When you are with your child, how present are you really—mentally and emotionally?

What moments or settings make it hardest for you to stay engaged?

RESOLVE:

Commit to one daily, distraction-free moment with your child—even if it's brief.

3. Emotional Presence in Difficult Moments

READ:

The chapter emphasizes listening, validation, patience, and calm during times of stress.

REFLECT:

How do you typically respond when your child is emotionally dysregulated or overwhelmed?

What emotional responses from your own childhood might be influencing how you show up now?

RESOLVE:

Choose one emotional skill to practice this week: listening, validating, slowing down, or staying calm.

4. Being Present as an Advocate and Educator

READ:

Fathers are called to be fully engaged in their child's education and development.

REFLECT:

How involved are you currently in your child's education, therapies, or IEP process?

What fears, assumptions, or time pressures might be holding you back?

RESOLVE:

Take one concrete step toward deeper educational involvement—attend, ask, read, or follow up.

5. Guiding the Heart

READ:

Spiritual presence is framed as guiding values, meaning, hope, and connection.

REFLECT:

What values or beliefs do you most want your child to absorb from you?

How do you personally find meaning or grounding during hard seasons?

RESOLVE:

Model one value intentionally this week—gratitude, patience, courage, faith, or hope.

Optional Close:

"Your presence—more than your provision—shapes your child's sense of safety, worth, and hope."

Chapter 5 | Father-to-Father Mentoring: Wisdom, Support, and Strength in Community

1. From Isolation to Brotherhood

READ:

The chapter names isolation as a common burden—
and mentoring as a way to relieve that.

REFLECT:

Where do you feel most alone in this journey (in the medical world,
the educational setting, your marriage, your emotions, your faith)?

What keeps you from reaching out—pride, time, fear, or "no one will get it"?

RESOLVE:

Identify one dad you will contact this week (text/call/message)
and take the first step toward connection.

2. The Power of Being Understood

READ:

Mentorship works because shared experience
creates empathy without explanation.

REFLECT:

What's something about your situation you're tired
of explaining to people who don't get it?

What would it feel like to talk to someone who
already understands the landscape?

RESOLVE:

Write down one sentence you'd be willing to share with a mentor or peer dad:

"The hardest part for me right now is _____."

3. Practical Wisdom That Saves Energy

READ:

Mentors don't replace professionals—but they can shorten the learning curve.

REFLECT:

Where do you most need "been there" guidance right now: health care, education/IEPs, behavior, work-life balance?

What mistake or time-waster do you wish you could avoid repeating?

RESOLVE:

Choose one area and seek one practical tip this week from a dad who's further down the road.

4. Permission to Be Vulnerable

READ:

Men often feel pressure to stay stoic; mentoring creates space to be real.

REFLECT:

What emotions do you hide most often—fear, sadness, anger, shame, loneliness?

What has stoicism cost you (stress, marriage tension, distance, burnout)?

RESOLVE:

Practice "strong and honest" by sharing one real feeling with a trusted person this week.

5. Becoming the Dad Who Gives Back

READ:

Mentoring is a long game: Today's mentee can become tomorrow's mentor.

REFLECT:

Who helped you most in your life, and what did they do that mattered?

What part of your journey could someday help another father feel less alone?

RESOLVE:

Take one step toward "giving back"—encourage a newer dad, share a resource, or offer to listen.

Optional Close:

"I don't have to carry this alone."

Chapter 6 | Self-Care for Dads: Prioritizing Your Well-Being to Better Serve Your Family

1. Self-Care Isn't Selfish

READ:

The chapter reframes self-care as the foundation for consistent fathering.

REFLECT:

When you hear "self-care," do you feel permission—or guilt? Why?

How has neglecting yourself shown up at home (irritability, exhaustion, numbness, resentment)?

RESOLVE:

Choose one self-care act you will do this week and treat it like a nonnegotiable appointment.

2. Your "Empty Cup" Warning Signs

READ:

Burnout creeps in when stress becomes constant and recovery disappears.

REFLECT:

What are your early warning signs that you're running on fumes?

What is your default coping strategy—and does it actually help long-term?

RESOLVE:

Pick one healthier outlet to use *before* you hit the wall (walk, workout, breathing, journaling, call a friend).

3. Physical Health as a Parenting Tool

READ:

Sleep, movement, and nutrition aren't vanity—they're capacity.

REFLECT:

Which one needs the most attention right now: sleep, movement, or eating well?

What is one small obstacle that keeps you from improving it (schedule, habits, stress, lack of plan)?

RESOLVE:

Make one specific upgrade for the next seven days (bedtime routine, short walk, healthier lunch, hydration).

4. Boundaries, Compartmentalizing, and the Courage to Ask for Help

READ:

The chapter challenges "testosterone poisoning"—the refusal to ask for directions.

REFLECT:

Where are you trying to do too much alone?

What's the story you tell yourself about asking for help—and is it true?

RESOLVE:

Ask for one kind of help this week (practical, emotional, professional, or peer support).

5. A Routine You Can Actually Keep

READ:

Consistency beats intensity; small rituals build resilience.

REFLECT:

What time of day is most realistic for a short self-care routine?

What would make it more likely to happen: a reminder, a buddy, or a tracker?

RESOLVE:

Create a simple "minimum viable routine" you can keep five days this week (ten minutes counts).

Optional Close:

"Taking care of myself is part of taking care of my family."

Chapter 7 | Respite and Renewal: The Importance of Taking Breaks Without Guilt

1. Respite Is a Strategy, Not an Escape

READ:

The chapter describes respite as "one step back, two steps forward."

REFLECT:

When you imagine taking a break, what feelings come up—relief, guilt, anxiety, or all of the above?

How might your family benefit if you were more rested and regulated?

RESOLVE:

Give yourself permission to schedule one break this week—even a small one.

2. Naming the Guilt

READ:

Guilt is often the biggest barrier to rest.

REFLECT:

What does your guilt say (e.g., "I should be doing more," "My child needs me," "I don't deserve a break")?

Where did you learn that message—family culture, masculinity expectations, or past experiences?

RESOLVE:

Replace guilt with a true statement you will repeat this week (e.g., *"Rest helps me show up better"*).

3. Building a Respite Plan That Fits Real Life

READ:

Respite can be minutes within a day, weekly, or scheduled care, but not just vacations.

REFLECT:

What kind of respite is most realistic right now: daily micro-breaks, weekly mini-breaks, or monthly meetups?

What's the most predictable window in your week you can protect?

RESOLVE:

Put one respite block on your calendar and protect it like an appointment.

4. Who Can You Trust with the Load?

READ:

Respite often requires a support network—people and programs.

REFLECT:

Who is truly in your "trusted circle" (family, friends, church, neighbors, other dads)?

What keeps you from asking them—fear of burdening others, safety concerns, or pride?

RESOLVE:

Identify one person or resource you will explore this week for respite support—and take one step (call, email, research).

5. Renewal That Actually Renews You

READ:

Breaks work best when they include activities that restore your body, mind, or joy.

REFLECT:

What genuinely renews you? Is it exercise, nature, solitude, hobbies, friends, faith, laughter?

What do you miss doing that used to make you feel like yourself?

RESOLVE:

Choose one renewing activity and do it this week— small is fine, but do it on purpose.

Optional Close:

"Respite isn't leaving my family—it's returning to them stronger."

Chapter 8 | Faith and Fatherhood: Spirituality as a Guide on the Special Needs Journey

1. Faith, Doubt, and Honest Questions

READ:

The chapter acknowledges that a diagnosis can trigger a crisis of faith—or deeper reflection.

REFLECT:

How has your child's diagnosis affected your beliefs about life, meaning, or fairness?

Where do you feel grounded, and where do you feel uncertain?

RESOLVE:

Give yourself permission to be honest about one question or doubt you've been carrying.

2. Meaning in the Midst of Challenge

READ:

Faith can help fathers seek purpose without needing all the answers.

REFLECT:

What phrases or beliefs have you used to cope with uncertainty? ("We'll cross that bridge," "Don't pre-worry")?

How have these challenges shaped you as a man or father?

RESOLVE:

Write or say one sentence that reflects the meaning you're finding *right now*—even if it's incomplete.

3. Spiritual Practices That Ground You

READ:

Spirituality can be practiced through prayer, worship, meditation, reading, nature, or reflection.

REFLECT:

What practices help you slow down, reflect, or
feel connected to something larger?

Which ones have you neglected during stressful seasons?

RESOLVE:

Reintroduce one simple practice this week—five minutes counts.

4. Faith, Community, and Support

READ:

Faith often grows stronger in community rather than isolation.

REFLECT:

Where do you feel supported spiritually? Or where do you feel alone?

What kind of community would feel authentic and safe for you?

RESOLVE:

Take one step toward connection. Attend, reach out, or
explore a group that aligns with your values.

5. Modeling Hope and Values

READ:

A father's spirituality often shapes the emotional climate of the family.

REFLECT:

What values do you hope your children absorb by watching how you live?

How do you model hope during hard seasons?

RESOLVE:

Intentionally model one value this week—gratitude,
compassion, perseverance, or grace.

Optional Close:

"I don't need all the answers to walk forward with purpose."

Chapter 9 | Siblings Matter: Balancing Attention and Love Across the Entire Family

1. Seeing All of Your Children

READ:

The chapter reminds fathers they are parents to *all* their children.

REFLECT:

Which child currently receives most of your time and attention—and why?

How might another child feel unseen or overlooked?

RESOLVE:

Schedule one intentional one-on-one time with a child who needs it.

2. The Hidden Load Carried by Siblings

READ:

Siblings may feel neglected or overly responsible or traumatized.

REFLECT:

How do your other children express stress, frustration, or withdrawal?

Have any taken on roles or maturity beyond their age?

RESOLVE:

Have one check-in conversation focused only on listening—no fixing.

3. Communication That Makes Room for Feelings

READ:

Open communication helps prevent resentment and confusion.

REFLECT:

How comfortable are your children expressing difficult emotions at home?

How do you typically respond when they do?

RESOLVE:

Practice reflective listening once this week: "What I hear you saying is..."

4. Inclusion Without Burden

READ:
Inclusion builds empathy, but siblings shouldn't become substitute parents.

REFLECT:
Where do your children help out willingly—
and where might it feel like too much?

How do you affirm their contributions without assigning responsibility?

RESOLVE:
Acknowledge one child's effort or strength out loud this week.

5. Building Bonds That Last a Lifetime

READ:
Sibling relationships often outlast parents.

REFLECT:
What memories or traditions help your children feel connected to one another?

How are you intentionally shaping sibling bonds?

RESOLVE:
Create or reinforce one shared family activity this week.

Optional Close:
"Every child in our family matters—fully and equally."

Chapter 10 | Family Leadership: Building a Strong, Healthy and Unified Household with Vision, Intent, and Values

1. Redefining Leadership at Home

READ:

Family leadership is about service, not control.

REFLECT:

When you hear the word "leader," what behaviors come to mind at home?

How does your family experience your leadership—calming, commanding, or missing in action?

RESOLVE:

Lead a situation by your example rather than with your words.

2. Vision and Values

READ:

A shared vision anchors families during uncertainty.

REFLECT:

What values define your family right now?

Are they spoken, written, or assumed?

RESOLVE:

Write down (or discuss) one core family value and what it looks like in action.

3. Intentional Time and Rituals

READ:

Strong families prioritize connection before convenience.

REFLECT:

What rituals bring your family together consistently?

Where have busyness or screens crept in?

RESOLVE:
Reinstate or protect one family ritual this week.

4. Communication and Collaboration

READ:
Open dialogue builds trust and resilience.

REFLECT:
How safe do family members feel sharing hard truths?

How do you handle disagreement at home?

RESOLVE:
Invite one collaborative conversation instead of making a unilateral decision.

5. Leading Through Crisis

READ:
Families need calm, compassionate leadership during storms.

REFLECT:
How do you respond emotionally during crisis—withdraw, control, or connect?

What does your family need most from you during uncertainty?

RESOLVE:
Practice emotional steadiness this week—pause, breathe, respond.

Optional Close:
"Leadership at home means taking care of those in my charge."

Chapter 11 | Mastermind Groups: Tapping into Collective Wisdom and Support

1. The Cost of Going It Alone

READ:

Isolation is one of the biggest threats to everyone and especially fathers of special needs kids.

REFLECT:

Where do you feel most alone right now?

What has isolation cost you—emotionally, relationally, or physically?

RESOLVE:

Admit (to yourself or others) one area where you need support.

2. The Power of Collective Wisdom

READ:

Mastermind groups multiply insight, clarity, and courage.

REFLECT:

What challenge could benefit from group perspective instead of solo problem-solving?

How open are you to learning from peers?

RESOLVE:

Share one challenge out loud this week—with someone you trust.

3. Accountability That Builds Momentum

READ:

Consistency and accountability fuel growth.

REFLECT:

Where do you start strong but fade without accountability?

How do you respond to encouragement versus pressure?

RESOLVE:

Name one goal and one accountability partner.

4. Commitment and Investment

READ:

Transformation requires time, presence, and commitment.

REFLECT:

What keeps you from committing to structured support—time, money, fear, habits?

What would change if you truly invested in yourself?

RESOLVE:

Decide one concrete next step: join, explore, or start a group.

5. From Participant to Leader

READ:

Every dad brings value to the circle.

REFLECT:

What life experience could help another father?

How might you contribute—not just receive?

RESOLVE:

Encourage or support one other dad this week.

Optional Close:

"You were never meant to carry this journey alone—shared wisdom, accountability, and brotherhood make fathers stronger and families more resilient."

Chapter 12 | IEPs, Setting and Accomplishing Goals, and Celebrating Wins, Large and Small

1. The IEP as a Starting Point

READ:

The chapter frames the IEP as a foundation—not a finish line.

REFLECT:

How do you currently feel when you walk into an IEP meeting—confident, anxious, frustrated, hopeful?

Where do you tend to stay silent when your voice might matter most?

RESOLVE:

Identify one specific way you will show up more intentionally at the next IEP meeting.

2. Goals Beyond the Classroom

READ:

True growth often happens outside school, in daily life.

REFLECT:

What life skills or personal goals matter most for your child right now?

How do those goals align with your child's interests and strengths?

RESOLVE:

Choose one meaningful, real-life goal to work on this month.

3. Measuring Progress Differently

READ:

Progress is often nonlinear and easy to overlook.

REFLECT:

What "small wins" might you be overlooking because you're focused on what's next?

How do you define success for your child today?

RESOLVE:

Commit to noticing and naming one small win each day this week.

4. The Power of Celebration

READ:

Celebration reinforces confidence, resilience, and identity.

REFLECT:

How was achievement acknowledged in your own childhood?

How do you currently celebrate effort—not just outcomes—with your child?

RESOLVE:

Create one simple, repeatable way to celebrate progress at home.

5. A Father's Steady Encouragement

READ:

A father's belief can outweigh systems, plans, and timelines.

REFLECT:

When has your belief in your child made a difference—even if no one else noticed?

What message does your child most need to hear from you right now?

RESOLVE:

Say those words—out loud—this week.

Optional Close:

"Every small step forward deserves to be seen."

Chapter 13 | Living in the Present: Thriving in the Circumstances You Didn't Expect

1. Accepting the Reality You're In

READ:

Acceptance is not surrender; it's the beginning of peace.

REFLECT:

Where are you still resisting the reality of your family's situation?

What emotions surface when you think about "what might have been"?

RESOLVE:

Name one aspect of your current reality you are ready to accept—without judgment.

2. Letting Go of Future Fear

READ:

Anxiety grows when we live too far ahead of today.

REFLECT:

What future worries consume the most mental energy for you?

How do those worries affect your presence with your family?

RESOLVE:

Practice redirecting your focus to one present-moment interaction each day.

3. Gratitude in Unexpected Places

READ:

Gratitude reshapes perspective.

REFLECT:

What moments of joy or connection happened recently that surprised you?

How has fatherhood changed what you're grateful for?

RESOLVE:

Write down three things you're grateful for each night this week.

4. Flexibility over Control

READ:

Thriving often requires releasing rigid expectations.

REFLECT:

Where do you struggle most when plans change or things go off script?

How does flexibility—or lack of it—affect your child?

RESOLVE:

Practice letting one plan go this week without frustration.

5. Choosing Perspective

READ:

You can't control circumstances, but you can control perspective.

REFLECT:

What perspective shift has helped you most on this journey so far?

What perspective might be holding you back?

RESOLVE:

Replace one negative internal narrative with a more compassionate one.

Optional Close:

"Today is enough."

Chapter 14 | The Unwavering Commitment: 24/7/365 Fatherhood and What It Really Takes

1. Understanding the Depth of Commitment

READ:

Fatherhood is a marathon, not a sprint.

REFLECT:

What does 24/7/365 commitment look like in your daily life?

Where do you feel most stretched or depleted?

RESOLVE:

Acknowledge one sacrifice you've made—and honor it without guilt.

2. Showing Up in the Ordinary

READ:

Everyday moments build trust and security.

REFLECT:

How present are you during daily routines like meals, homework, or bedtime?

What small moments do you want your child to remember?

RESOLVE:

Choose one daily routine to engage in more fully this week.

3. The Toll on Mind and Body

READ:

Unwavering commitment requires sustainability.

REFLECT:

Which stressors impact you most right now—financial, emotional, relational, physical?

How do you typically cope?

RESOLVE:

Commit to one self-care or support action this week—without apology.

4. Resilience Through Adversity

READ:

Resilience grows through challenges, not despite them.

REFLECT:

What challenges have shaped you into a stronger father?

How do you model resilience for your child?

RESOLVE:

Reframe one ongoing challenge as a growth opportunity.

5. Never Giving Up

READ:

Persistence sends a powerful message to your child.

REFLECT:

What does "never giving up" look like for you right now?

Who or what inspires you to keep going?

RESOLVE:

Recommit—privately or publicly—to staying the course.

Optional Close:

"I am here—always."

Chapter 15 | Fostering Independence and Self-Sufficiency: Helping Your Child Build Confidence, Find Purpose, and Gain Employment

1. Redefining Independence

READ:

Independence is about dignity, not distance.

REFLECT:

What does independence mean for your child specifically?

Where do you tend to step in too quickly?

RESOLVE:

Identify one task your child can do with less help.

2. Building Confidence Through Responsibility

READ:

Competence builds confidence.

REFLECT:

What responsibilities does your child already handle well?

How do you communicate belief in their abilities?

RESOLVE:

Gradually fade support in one area this month.

3. Teaching Problem-Solving and Self-Advocacy

READ:

Decision-making skills are as important as functional skills.

REFLECT:

How often do you invite your child into decision-making?

How do you model problem-solving in your own life?

RESOLVE:

"Think out loud" during one real-life decision this week.

4. Discovering Purpose and Passion

READ:

Purpose fuels motivation and joy.

REFLECT:

What activities light your child up?

How can those interests translate into contribution in your home or community or work?

RESOLVE:

Explore one new experience aligned with your child's interests.

5. Preparing for Adulthood—Together

READ:

Independence is a lifelong process.

REFLECT:

What adult life skills feel most urgent right now?

Who can help support your child's growth beyond your family?

RESOLVE:

Take one concrete step toward your child's future independence.

Optional Close:

"True independence grows when we replace doing for our children with believing in them, equipping them, and walking alongside them toward a life of dignity and purpose."

Chapter 16 | Protecting Your Family: The Importance of Estate and Financial Planning

1. Facing the Question We All Carry

READ:

"What happens to my child when I'm gone?"

REFLECT:

What emotions come up for you when you think about your child's future without you?

What has delayed or complicated planning for your family so far?

RESOLVE:

Write down one concrete planning question you're ready to address.

2. Love Translated into Structure

READ:

Planning is not paperwork—it's protection.

REFLECT:

How do you currently express love through preparation and responsibility?

What would peace of mind look like for you and your spouse or partner?

RESOLVE:

Commit to one planning step you will take in the next thirty days.

3. Avoiding Unintended Harm

READ:

Well-meaning decisions can accidentally jeopardize benefits.

REFLECT:

Were you aware of how inheritances or beneficiary designations could affect SSI or Medicaid?

Who else in your family (grandparents, siblings) may need education on this topic?

RESOLVE:

Identify one person with whom you need to have a planning conversation.

4. Guardianship, Trust, and Team

READ:

No father plans alone.

REFLECT:

Who do you trust to care for your child if you cannot?

What qualities matter most in a future guardian, conservator, or trustee?

RESOLVE:

Begin a written list of potential guardians/conservators or advocates.

5. Legacy Beyond Your Lifetime

READ:

Planning extends your fatherhood forward.

REFLECT:

How does responsible planning reflect your values as a dad?

What legacy do you want your planning decisions to communicate?

RESOLVE:

Take one action this week that honors your role as protector.

Optional Close:

"Planning today is an act of love tomorrow."

Chapter 17 | Dads Raising Children with Autism: Navigating a Unique Path with Love and Patience

1. Seeing the Individual, Not the Label

READ:

"If you've met one person with autism, you've met one person with autism."

REFLECT:

How has your understanding of autism evolved over time?

Where have you learned the most—professionals or lived experience?

RESOLVE:

Commit to learning directly from one autistic self-advocate this month.

2. Patience as a Daily Practice

READ:

Patience creates safety.

REFLECT:

What situations most test your patience as a father?

How does your child respond when you remain calm?

RESOLVE:

Identify one trigger and plan how you'll respond differently next time.

3. Communication That Respects Difference

READ:

Communication is connection.

REFLECT:

How does your child best communicate stress, joy, or needs?

Where could you adjust your communication style?

RESOLVE:

Practice one new communication strategy this week.

4. Celebrating Small Wins

READ:

Progress often comes quietly.

REFLECT:

What recent progress deserves more recognition?

How do celebrations affect your child's confidence?

RESOLVE:

Create a simple ritual to acknowledge effort.

5. Walking Beside, Not Ahead

READ:

This is your child's path—not a race.

REFLECT:

Where are you tempted to compare your child to others?

What does unconditional support look like today?

RESOLVE:

Release one comparison and replace it with encouragement.

Optional Close:

"Different paths still lead to meaningful lives."

Chapter 18 | Supporting Children with Down Syndrome: Focusing on Abilities, Not Limitations

1. Redefining What's Possible

READ:

Abilities deserve the spotlight.

REFLECT:

What strengths in your child bring you the most joy?

How often do you speak about abilities rather than limitations?

RESOLVE:

Intentionally name one strength to your child this week.

2. Building Confidence Through Independence

READ:

Confidence grows through doing.

REFLECT:

Where does your child want more independence?

Where might you be helping too much?

RESOLVE:

Step back slightly in one area and allow growth.

3. Advocacy as Fatherhood

READ:

Your voice matters.

REFLECT:

Where have you had to advocate hardest for your child?

What fears hold you back from speaking up?

RESOLVE:

Prepare for your next advocacy moment with clarity and courage.

4. Community and Belonging

READ:

No family thrives alone.

REFLECT:

What communities have supported your journey?

Where do you need deeper connection?

RESOLVE:

Reach out to one family or organization this month.

5. Celebrating the Journey

READ:

Joy is a form of resilience.

REFLECT:

How do you celebrate effort, not just outcomes?

What traditions could reinforce pride and belonging?

RESOLVE:

Start one new celebration tradition at home.

Optional Close:

"Different abilities. Equal dignity."

Chapter 19 | Rare Diseases and Resilience: Adapting to the Unknown with Courage

1. Living with Uncertainty

READ:

Rare diseases redefine certainty.

REFLECT:

What uncertainty weighs heaviest on you right now?

How has not knowing changed you?

RESOLVE:

Identify one thing you can control today.

2. Knowledge as Power

READ:

Information can bring clarity—or complexity.

REFLECT:

How did diagnosis (or lack of one) affect your family?

What fears surround genetic testing or medical decisions?

RESOLVE:

Write down questions you need answered by a professional.

3. Emotional Resilience

READ:

Strength grows under pressure.

REFLECT:

How do you process fear, grief, or exhaustion?

Who supports you emotionally?

RESOLVE:

Ask for help in one specific way this week.

4. Purpose Through Advocacy

READ:

Pain can fuel purpose.

REFLECT:

How has your experience shaped your values?

Where might your story help others?

RESOLVE:

Share your story—or listen to another family's.

5. Redefining Strength

READ:

Resilience is learned.

REFLECT:

What has this journey taught you about courage?

How has your child strengthened you?

RESOLVE:

Name one way you will honor that resilience.

Optional Close:

"Resilience is built, not inherited."

Chapter 20 | Cerebral Palsy and Strength: Overcoming Challenges with Determination

1. Seeing Ability First

READ:

CP does not define potential.

REFLECT:

How does your child define themselves?

How do you reinforce identity beyond diagnosis?

RESOLVE:

Affirm your child's identity this week—clearly and confidently.

2. Supporting Physical Challenges

READ:

Movement may look different—but progress is real.

REFLECT:

What therapies or tools have made the biggest difference?

How do you respond when progress is slow?

RESOLVE:

Celebrate effort, not speed.

3. Emotional Strength

READ:

Confidence grows through encouragement.

REFLECT:

How does your child respond to praise?

Where might they need more affirmation?

RESOLVE:

Intentionally praise persistence this week.

4. Education and Opportunity

READ:

Access creates possibility.

REFLECT:

How well does your child's educational plan serve them?

Where could advocacy improve outcomes?

RESOLVE:

Prepare for your next school conversation with intention.

5. The Long View

READ:

Determination compounds over time.

REFLECT:

What dreams does your child hold for the future?

How can you help remove one barrier?

RESOLVE:

Take one step toward that future today.

Optional Close:

"Strength is measured by persistence."

Chapter 21 | The Legacy of Fatherhood: Leaving a Lasting Impact on Your Family and Community

1. Defining Legacy

READ:

Legacy is lived, not left.

REFLECT:

What lessons did you inherit from your own father?

Which do you want to pass on—and which to break?

RESOLVE:

Choose one value you want your children to remember you for.

2. Presence over Perfection

READ:

Presence changes everything.

REFLECT:

Where does distraction pull you away most?

When has your presence mattered more than anything else?

RESOLVE:

Be fully present for one meaningful moment this week.

3. Modeling Values Daily

READ:

Children learn by watching.

REFLECT:

What behaviors are you modeling unintentionally?

How do you handle mistakes at home?

RESOLVE:

Model accountability through one apology or repair.

4. Influence Beyond the Home

READ:

Fathers shape communities.

REFLECT:

Who have you influenced without realizing it?

How can your example encourage other dads?

RESOLVE:

Encourage one father this month.

5. What Will Matter Most

READ:

Legacy outlives achievements.

REFLECT:

What do you hope your children say about you someday?

Are your current priorities aligned with that hope?

RESOLVE:

Make one choice today that honors the legacy you want.

Optional Close:

"Your legacy is not what you leave for your children. It is what you leave in them."

This workbook is a companion, not a finish line. Return to it as often as needed. Growth happens through presence, consistency, and compassion.

This curriculum is a good starting point to give you a sense of who you are as a dad, and who you could be. Being a father is a lifetime commitment, and one of the ways you can keep your commitment strong is to connect with other dads and organizations that provide support.

The Special Fathers Network provides a wide range of practical resources and timely assistance for dads seeking advice. The 21st Century Dads Foundation website at www.21stCenturyDads.org provides access to more than four hundred *SFN Dad To Dad Podcast* episodes, more than one hundred books on fathering, special needs, leadership, and more. The site is also a portal for requesting an SFN Mentor Father or volunteering to become one of more than nine hundred SFN Mentor Fathers. You'll also be able to learn about the SFN Mastermind Group program.

For ongoing information, you can subscribe to the weekly 21st Century Dads e-Newsletter, for FREE at www.21stCenturyDads.org.

Appendix A: Books and 21CD Resources

Here are some other titles by David Hirsch:

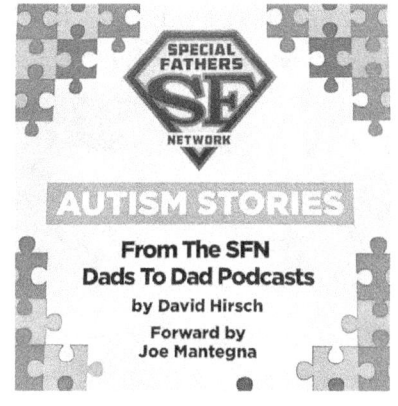
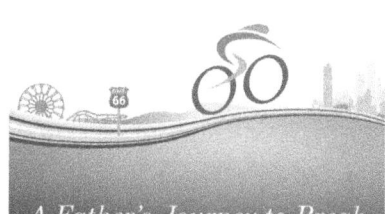
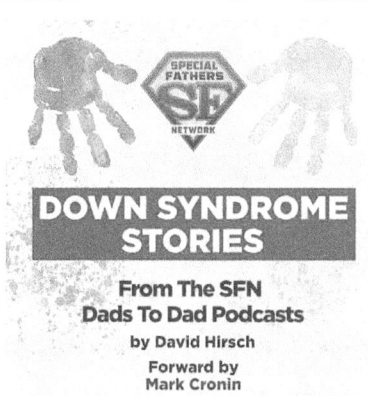
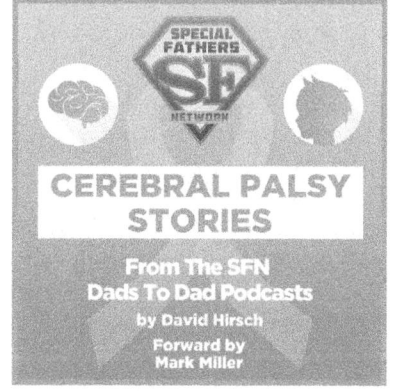
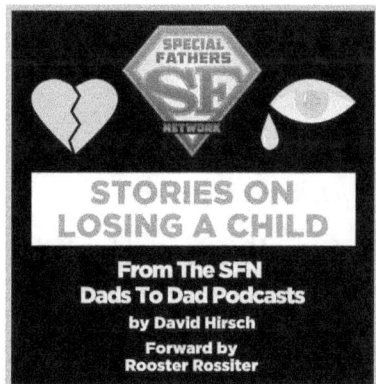
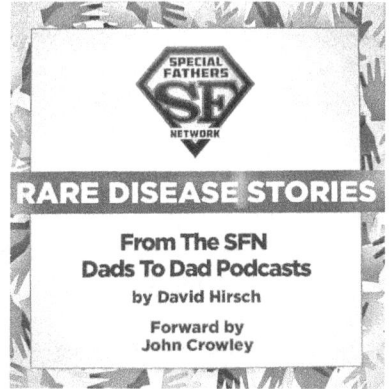

The initial SFN Mastermind Group started meeting in July 2020 during the peak of COVID-19. The following is a list of books read and the authors who did Zoom calls with the initial and subsequent SFN Mastermind Group dads once every two months (in the chronological order the books were read). *Note:* virtually everyone of these books were authored by SFN Mentor Fathers or those who did interviews for the *SFN Dad To Dad Podcast*. We're very proud of the depth of knowledge within the Special Fathers Network.

Another Kind of Courage: God's Design for Fathers of Families Affected by Disability by Doug Maza and Steve Bundy

Be a Better Parent: 10 Strategies for Being the Best You Can Be for Your Child by Dr. Bob Franks

Keep It Together Man: For Dads with a Special Kid by Rick Daynes

The Ultimate Gift by Jim Stovall

Secrets of the Bulletproof Spirit: How to Bounce Back from Life's Hardest Hits by Azim Khamisa

The Leader Within Us: Mindset, Principles and Tools for a Life by Design by Warren Rustand

Financial Freedom for Special Needs Families: 9 Building Blocks to Reduce Stress, Preserve Benefits, and Create a Fulfilling Future by Rob Wrubel

Smart Leadership: Four Simple Choices to Scale Your Impact by Mark Miller

Thinking in Pictures: My Life with Autism by Dr. Temple Grandin

The Voice of Victory: One Man's Journey to Freedom Through Healing & Forgiveness by Wayne Messmer

The Fun Master: A Memoir by Jeff Seitzer

One More Step: Making the Impossible Possible by Bonner Paddock

Adversitology: Overcoming Adversity When You're Hanging by a Thread by Frank McKinney

Aspertools: The Practical Guide for Understanding and Embracing Asperger's, Autism Spectrum Disorders and Neurodiversity by Dr. Hackie Reitman

APPENDIX A: BOOKS AND 21CD RESOURCES

Angel for Higher by Robert Hendershot

Zero to Hero: From Bullied Kid to Warrior by Allen Lynch

A View from the Top: Living a Life of Significance by Aaron Walker

What I Wish I Knew Back Then: A Physical Therapist and Mother's Perspective of Raising Her Child with Cerebral Palsy by Marsh Naidoo

The Gift I Was Given: The Journey of a Caregiver Through the Stages of What Now? Why Me? & Ah Ha! by Mary Anne Ehlert

Aspire: How to Create Your Own Reality and Alter Your DNA by Frank McKinney

A Long Walk Down a Winding Road: Small Steps, Challenges, and Triumphs Through an Autistic Lens by Sam Farmer

Fix Your B.S. (Belief Systems) by Dr. Greg Pursley

Lovin' with Grit & Grace: Straight-Talk About Romance, Sex, Fun and the Tough Stuff Too by Jesse Ronne

Parenting Beyond Power: How to Use Connection and Collaboration to Transform Your Family—and the World by Jen Lumanlan

How to Build a Thriving Marriage as You Care for Children with Disability by Kristin & Todd Evans

Seeing Ability: Finding Your Path in Parenting a Child with Special Needs by Jim Littlefield-Dalmares

No Greatness Without Goodness: How a Father's Love Changed a Company & Sparked a Movement by Randy Lewis

The Doman Method: From Special Needs to Wellness by Spencer Doman

Dads Like Us: Raising a Child with Disabilities by Steve Harris

**For more suggested reading, visit
https://21stcenturydads.org/book-recommendations/
or scan the QR code.**

SFN DAD To Dad Podcast Guests

1. Tony Oommen
2. Randy Lewis
3. Skip Gianopulos
4. Jim Elliott
5. Joe Mantegna
6. Paul Gianni
7. Clayton Frech
8. Jeff Aeder
9. Scott Sowers
10. Bob Roybal
11. Dick Hoyt
12. Shanne Sowards
14. Jim Mueller
15. Dan Marquardt
16. Rob Gorski
17. Mark Cronin
18. Tom Landis
19. Brian Page
20. Gene Andrasco
21. Dan McNeil
22. Adam Levy
23. Joe Ciriano
24. Peter Morici
25. Rabbi Bradley Shavit Artson
26. David Friedman
27. Brian Rubin
28. Joe Butler
29. Rooster Rossiter
30. Paul Miller
31. Kris Kazian
32. Bob Bjerkaas
33. Lee Jorwic
34. Steve Bundy
35. Peter Bell
36. Dave Elsinger
37. Matt Mooney
38. Josh Jacobs
39. Mark Maguire
40. Brent Chase
41. Stacy Tetschner
42. Paul Koza
43. Charles Ware
44. Tom Delaney
45. Rick Daynes
46. Jon Ebersole
47. Seth Keiffer
48. Gregg Chalmers
49. Haki Nkrumah
50. Rick Bovell
51. Bo Bigelow
52. John Shouse
53. Steve Duffley
54. Rich Gathro
55. Becky Davidson
56. Wayne Messmer
57. Tim Kuck
58. Bob Mendez
59. Sean Farrell
60. Martin Cuevas
61. Jason Lehmbeck
62. John Wagner
63. Kelly Moynihan
64. Shane Lee
65. John Felageller
66. Jerry Castro
67. Jim Abrahams
68. John Dodd
69. Tom Costello
70. Dan Tepperman
71. John Crowley
72. Shane Sondergeld
73. Jim Rigg
74. Cory Estby
75. Mark Paterson
76. Jeff Katz
77. Michael Kohler
78. Chad Johnson
79. John Kimec
80. Steve Mogul
81. Jude Morrow
82. Josh Avis
83. John Heckert
84. Special Moments
85. Don Garner
86. Dan Morrissey
87. Jaun Vagilenty
88. Mark O'Halloran
89. On Losing a Child
90. Hackie Reitman
91. Rob Wrubel
92. Down Syndrome
93. Sam Rodriguez
94. Jarell Roach
95. Joe Lofino
96. Miguel Cervantes
97. Adaptive Sports
98. David Hall
99. Lawrence Fung
100. Doron Almog
101. Ben Satterfield
102. Robert Blackwell
103. Jonathan McGuire
104. Stephen Grcevich
105. Richard Shuster
106. Jose Velasco
107. Mike Carmody
108. Nik Nikic
109. Brian & Allen Lynch
110. Stephen Drum
111. Roddy Vannoy
112. Jack Levin
113. Jim Vaselopulos
114. Nathan Woerner
115. Daniel DeFabio
116. Daniel DeFabio
117. Chris LaFriniare
118. Dwayne Wiseman
119. Al Feria
120. Mark Arnold
121. Bruce Hearey
122. Stephen "Doc" Hunsley
123. Alex Lyubelsky
124. Lon Haldeman
125. Bill Danko
126. Blair Cornell
127. Bob Franks
128. Evan Spotswood
129. Michael Striegl
130. Phil Irwin
131. Phil Irwin
132. Casey Parks
133. Rob Johnson
134. James Mack
135. Tony Gayle
136. Tony Gayle
137. Rob Kenney
138. Don Raineri
139. Lyle Liechty
140. Chris Wade
141. Rob Harris
142. Warren Rustand
143. Warren Rustand
144. Andy McCall
145. Jeremy Kredlo
146. Larry Kaufman
147. Azim Khamisa
148. Ruslan Vasyutin
149. Felimon Hernandez
150. Mitch Gardner
151. Rolando Lopez
152. Jeremy Meinhardt
153. Ray Morris
154. Shane Madden
155. Jeff Johnson
156. Kyle Malone
157. Mary Anne Ehlert
158. Tom Hamilton
159. Ray Arata
160. Osman Arain
161. Chris Jones
162. Bailey Pratt
163. Jim Stovall
164. Brian Martin
165. Chad Lunt
166. Taruj Ali
167. Mike Ensminger
168. John Rosemond
169. Frederick Jefferson
170. Paul Mannino
171. Dan Habib
172. Marilyn York
173. Greg Hubert
174. Jeremy Knakmuhs
175. Harsha Rajasimha
176. Mark Huhtanen
177. Louis Geigerman
178. Gary Martinez
179. Scott Newport
180. Josh Poynter
181. Don "DJ" Joss
182. John DeGarmo
183. Jason Hsieh
184. Ágúst Kristmanns
185. Lenn Boston
186. Mark Miller
187. Edgar Pacheco
188. Tom D'Amato
189. Amjad Farah
190. Shandra Cubin
191. Ruslan Vasyutin
192. Eliya Stromberg
193. Miguel Sancho
194. Al Freedman
195. Susanna Peace-Lovell
196. Spela Mirosevic
197. Josh LaBelle
198. Jeremiah Kuria
199. Damion Navarro
200. Bill Strickland
201. Duncan Keya
202. Catherine Whitcher
203. Riana Milne
204. Mike Graglia
205. Justin DeVault
206. Chris Velona
207. Sarah Putt
208. Doug Robb
209. Shayne Gaffney
210. Kalman Samuels
211. Adam Bleakney, Amanda McGrory & Brian Siemann
212. Joe Lang
213. Eric Endlich
214. Jesse Hohn & Toby Brown
215. Jim Mullen
216. Sanath Kumar
217. Doug Noll
218. Pete Hixson
219. Jessica & Chris Patay
220. Anju Usman
221. Dr. John DeMartini
222. Christian Sakamoto
223. Michael DeLeon
224. Stewart Perriliat
225. Ron Janowczyk
226. Owen Marcus
227. Joshua Carrigg
228. Dr. Judson Brandeis
229. Shawn Francis & Brian Altounian
230. Bonner Paddock Rinn
231. Nelson Rascon
232. David Barth
233. Michelle Watson-Canfield
234. Michelle Watson-Canfield
235. David Geslak
236. Temple Grandin
237. Matt Bando
238. Ian Todd

239. Chris Brewster
240. Ron Sandison
241. Corey Ferguson
242. Cole Galloway
243. Christian Paddock
244. Joel Liestman
245. Marsh Naidoo
246. Paul Peterangelo
247. Jeff Seitzer
248. Olivier Bernier
249. Robert Hendershot
250. Tom Dreesen
251. Tom Dreesen
252. Bob West
253. Francis Arana
254. Jesse White
255. Steve Chatman
256. Jahmeer Reynolds
257. David Ross
258. Ben Mattlin
259. Ryan Wolfe
260. Frank McKinney
261. Frank McKinney
262. Adam Terry
263. Hutch Matteson
264. Siggi Thorseinn-Gudmunsson
265. Krista Mason
266. Dan Redfield
267. Jeff Zaugg
268. Tony Brescia
269. Eric Jorgensen
270. Eric Swithin
271. Medard Laz
272. Medard Laz
273. Rob Billerbeck
274. Brady Murray
275. Nate Boltz
276. Paul Carroll
277. Gus Aguilera
278. Adam Birchmeier
279. Tim Coughlin
280. Sara Glofcheskie
281. Jeff Wickersham
282. Brad Serot
283. Dan Feshbach
284. Will Derouen
285. Florence Ann Romano
286. Faye Simon-Harac
287. Bob Bourke
288. Jonathan Eig
289. James Myles
290. Graham Caldow
291. Dave Jereb
292. Allan Shedlin
293. Bob Manganelli
294. Bob Manganelli
295. Eric Nixon
296. Adam Goldman
297. Keith Harris
298. Keith Harris
299. Steve Thomas
300. Anniversary Episode
301. Jonathan Bennett
302. Gabe Perna
303. Allan Turner
304. Greg Pursley
305. Gary Rabine
306. Marc Moschetto
307. John Borling
308. Rich Gathro
309. Jon Ghahate
310. Matthew Rehbein
311. Jordan Jankus
312. Jeff Johnson
313. Paul Briggs
314. John Shouse
315. Leonardo Cespedes
316. Jon Heckert
317. Noel Fernández Collett
318. Shane Madden
319. Kelley Coleman
320. Ian Todd
321. Sam Farmer
322. Tony Brescia
323. Al Malavolti
324. Matt Bando
325. Al Malavolti
326. Jason Hsieh
327. Scott Maulsby
328. Tim Coughlin
329. Dave Van Doorn
330. Jordan Jankus
331. Alvin Green
332. John Fela
333. Mazi Keyghobadi
334. Tom Costello
335. DeAndrae Hinton
336. Joe Lofino
337. Jonathan Polin
338. Nathan Woerner
339. Bill Walters
340. MG Retreat Recap
341. Nate Plasman
342. Ágúst Kristmanns
343. Chris Mallette
344. Todd Evans
345. Chris Hunter
346. Ruslan Vasyutin
347. Tony Bombacino
348. Mike Abramowitz
349. Andrew Bustamante
350. Dana Lange
351. Wayne & Reena Friedman
352. Todd Evans
353. Tom Parro
354. Dennis Watkins
355. Phillip Koontz
356. Tieal Bishop
357. Craig Parks
358. Emma Livingstone
359. Look Back on 2024
360. Jessica Ronne
361. Scott MacGregor
362. Michael McManus
363. Jason Tuttle
364. Alfred Niwagaba
365. Isaac Jean-Paul
366. James Burch
367. Sebastien Pelletier
368. Tim Kane
369. Kirby Rabalais
370. Rady Johnson
371. Jen Lumanlan
372. Jason Bechtold
373. Michael Pereira
374. Eli Pierce
375. Jamiel Owens
376. Patrick Schwarz
377. Jim Littlefield-Dalmares
378. Leon Logothetis
379. Rebekah Taussig
380. Spencer Doman
381. Rick Bolle
382. Peter Gerhardt
383. Peter Gerhardt
384. Steve Harris
385. Steve Harris
386. Paul Collins
387. Randy Pierce
388. Randy Pierce
389. Robert Naseef
390. Tom Sander
391. Chris Losacco
392. Dion Chavis
393. Mike Rinaldi
394. Jelani Memory
395. Mark Reinfeld
396. Olivier Cortambert
397. Daryl Potter
398. Luba Patlakh
399. Casey Stubbs
400. Anniversary Issue
401. Greg Corey
402. David Apple
403. Swapna Sasidharan
404. Tom Chibucos
405. JP Klop
406. Dave Tolmie & Tumsifu Munuo
407. Jeff Wallis
408. Eric Freund
409. Nick & Cole Massie
410. John O'Leary
411. John O'Leary
412. Mike Kinner
413. Hugh Hempel
414. Hugh Hempel
415. Brad Meshell
416. Christian Pache
417. Patton Dodd
418. Mike Griffiths
419. Matt Shepherd
420. Rob Floyd

SFN Mastermind Group Dads

Matt Bando
Jason Bechtold
Bob Blameuser
Tony Bombacino
Tony Brescia
Tom Costello
Timothy Coughlin
Danny Dingeldein
Todd Evans
John Fela
Al Feria
Rich Gathro

Steve Harris
Jon Heckert
David Hirsch
Jordan Jankus
Jeff Johnson
Mazi Keyghobadi
Grant Krieg
Ágúst Kristmanns
Dana Lange
Chris Locasso
Joe Lofino
Alex Lyubelsky

Shane Madden
Chris Mallette
Rob McAfee
Mike McIntyre
Eli Pierce
Nate Plasman
David Porter
Kirby Rabalais
Matthew Rehbein
Brian Rouse
Nuwan Samaraweara
David Schwendtner

Jeff Seitzer
John Shouse
Nathan Simpson
Baskar Sriinvason
Ian Todd
Juan Vaglienty
Ruslan Vasyutin
Eric Williams
Nathan Woerner

SFN Mastermind Group Statement of Intent

The following is the SFN Mastermind Group Statement of Intent that each dads signs and pledges to adhere to. We welcome you to attend a weekly SFN Mastermind Group for one month and at no cost of obligation to see if this is a good fit for you. It might just transform your life, as it has done for so many others.

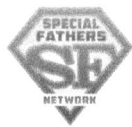

SFN Mastermind Group
Statement of Intent

The SFN mastermind Group is for men committed to being the absolute best dad and husband they can be. Members are committed to improving their situation while simultaneously assisting others to do the same. The overarching objective is to stay physically, emotionally and spiritually fit.

As a SFN Mastermind Group dad, I agree to the following:

- To Attend the weekly meetings,
- To Respect the opinions of others,
- To Share openly in the discussions,
- To Honor the confidentiality of the information discussed,
- To Meet my financial commitment of $200/month (or whatever I can afford)
- To Read the books, be prepared for the discussions and attend the author Zooms,
- To Serve as Dad-In-the-Middle every 4-5 weeks,
- To Facilitate the weekly meetings every 6-8 weeks,
- To Substitute for fellow members when asked,
- To Be Honest and Authentic, and
- To Have Fun.

_____   _____
Signature   Date

Please submit to: RSVP@21stCenturyDads.org

21st Century Dads Fatherhood Self-Assessment

The 21CD Fathering Self-Assessment Tool

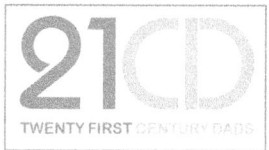

We spend time based on our own sense of priorities. For men with families the basic tug-of-war for time is between **family** and **work**.

When asked, most men would say their family is the most important aspect of their lives. While fathering, like mothering, doesn't come with a handbook, there are two primary obstacles to becoming a better father: **time** and **awareness**.

Congratulations for taking the time to take this self-assessment and develop a greater awareness for improving your fathering. Being a Great Dad is no more than being a great leader within your family. The process starts with figuring out where you are and then charting a path to where you want to be. This self-assessment tool is meant to be a starting point.

Instructions: answer each of these questions candidly and honestly. Remember, you are self scoring this assessment and you are doing this for your own benefit. The purpose is to identify where you are today, not where you want to be.

This assessment is divided into four categories: **Financial**, **Physical**, **Emotional**, and **Spiritual**. Score yourself on a scale of 0 to 5 using the following ratings:

0 - Not Applicable	1 - Never	2 - Rarely	3 - Periodically	4 - Frequently	5 - Always

Financial –
1. Do you talk about saving and investing with your children? 0 1 2 3 4 5
2. Do you provide your children with an allowance? 0 1 2 3 4 5
3. Do you play games like Monopoly and Cashflow with your children? 0 1 2 3 4 5
4. Do you provide 100% of your family's weekly financial support? 0 1 2 3 4 5
5. Do you involve your children with donations to charities? 0 1 2 3 4 5
6. Do you read financial publications (i.e. WSJ, Business Week, Forbes, etc.)? 0 1 2 3 4 5
TOTAL_____

Physical –
1. Do you exercise on a daily basis? 0 1 2 3 4 5
2. Do you spend at least 2 hours a day with your children? 0 1 2 3 4 5
3. Do you eat dinner with your children? 0 1 2 3 4 5
4. Do you interact with your children's teachers? 0 1 2 3 4 5
5. Do you talk with the parents of your children's friends? 0 1 2 3 4 5
6. Do you hug your kids on a daily basis? 0 1 2 3 4 5
7. Do you help your children with their homework? 0 1 2 3 4 5
8. Do you avoid habits or actions you want your children to avoid (i.e. drugs, alcohol, and smoking)? 0 1 2 3 4 5
TOTAL_____

Emotional –
1. Do you tell your kids daily that you love them? 0 1 2 3 4 5
2. Do you talk with your kids about their hopes and dreams? 0 1 2 3 4 5
3. Do you talk with your kids about their fears and concerns? 0 1 2 3 4 5
4. Do you handle crises in a calm manner without striking your kids or raising your voice? 0 1 2 3 4 5
5. Do you show respect to the mother of your children? 0 1 2 3 4 5
6. Do you talk with your parents on a weekly basis? 0 1 2 3 4 5
TOTAL_____

Spiritual –
1. Do you read the bible on a daily basis? 0 1 2 3 4 5
2. Do you meet weekly with a bible study group? 0 1 2 3 4 5
3. Do you attend Church/Synagogue/Mosque weekly with your children? 0 1 2 3 4 5
4. Do you pray with your kids? 0 1 2 3 4 5
5. Do you talk with you children about age appropriate faith based issues
   (i.e. telling the truth, respecting others, non-violence, etc.)? 0 1 2 3 4 5
6. Do you tithe your earnings? 0 1 2 3 4 5
TOTAL_____

Appendix B: A Primer of Additional Resources for Parents Raising Children with Special Needs and Disabilities

This appendix serves as a primer of resources available to parents raising children with special needs and disabilities. These resources include websites, organizations, support groups, and educational tools designed to assist families in navigating the challenges and opportunities associated with special needs parenting. The resources are categorized by type for easy reference.

1. National and International Organizations

United States
- **Biotechnology Innovation Organization (BIO)**
  - https://www.bio.org/
  - The world's largest advocacy organization representing the biotechnology industry—including biotech companies, academic and research institutions, state biotech centers, and related organizations. It works to promote innovation in health-care, agricultural, industrial, and environmental biotech, advocates for public policy that supports scientific progress, and hosts major industry events such as the BIO International Convention.
- **National Parent Center on Transition and Employment**
  - www.parentcenterhub.org
  - Provides resources to help parents navigate the transition to adulthood for children with disabilities.
- **Special Needs Alliance**
  - www.specialneedsalliance.org
  - A national organization of attorneys dedicated to assisting families of individuals with disabilities in planning for their future.
- **American Association on Intellectual and Developmental Disabilities (AAIDD)**
  - www.aaidd.org
  - Provides resources and information on intellectual and developmental disabilities, including research and advocacy.
- **Autism Society**
  - autismsociety.org
  - A national organization dedicated to supporting individuals with autism and their families through education, advocacy, and services.
- **National Down Syndrome Society (NDSS)**
  - www.ndss.org
  - Provides resources and support for individuals with Down syndrome and their families.
- **Cerebral Palsy Foundation**
  - www.cerebralpalsyfoundation.org
  - Offers resources, support, and information for families affected by cerebral palsy.

International
- **International Clearinghouse on Children with Disabilities (ICCD)**
  - www.iccd.com
  - Provides resources and information on children with disabilities around the globe.
- **Down Syndrome International**
  - www.ds-int.org
  - An organization promoting the rights of individuals with Down syndrome worldwide.
- **Autism-Europe**
  - www.autismeurope.org
  - A European organization that advocates for the rights and well-being of individuals with autism.

2. Support Groups and Networks

United States
- **Parent to Parent USA**
  - www.p2pusa.org
  - A national network of organizations providing support through connections with other parents.
- **The Arc**
  - www.thearc.org
  - A national organization advocating for and supporting individuals with intellectual and developmental disabilities.
- **National Federation of Families**
  - www.ffcmh.org
  - Provides support, education, and advocacy for families of children with mental health needs.

International
- **Rare Disease International (RDI)**
  - www.rarediseasesinternational.org
  - Supports individuals with rare diseases and their families through advocacy and awareness.
- **Family Voices**
  - www.familyvoices.org
  - A national organization of families advocating for health care for children and youth with special health-care needs.

3. Educational Resources and Toolkits

United States
- **Council for Exceptional Children (CEC)**
  - www.exceptionalchildren.org
  - Provides resources for educators, parents, and advocates in the field of special education.
- **National Center for Learning Disabilities (NCLD)**
  - www.ncld.org
  - Offers resources for understanding and supporting children with learning disabilities.

- **KidsHealth**
  - www.kidshealth.org
  - Provides health and development information for children, including resources on special needs.

International
- **UNESCO's Inclusive Education**
  - www.unesco.org/en/inclusion-education
  - Offers resources and guidance for inclusive education practices worldwide.
- **European Agency for Special Needs and Inclusive Education**
  - www.european-agency.org
  - Provides resources and research on inclusive education practices across Europe.

4. Therapeutic and Health Resources

United States
- **American Speech-Language-Hearing Association (ASHA)**
  - www.asha.org
  - Provides resources for speech and language therapy for children with communication disorders.
- **American Occupational Therapy Association (AOTA)**
  - www.aota.org
  - Offers resources related to occupational therapy for children with disabilities.
- **National Autism Association**
  - www.nationalautismassociation.org
  - Provides resources and support for families affected by autism, including safety and advocacy information.

International
- **World Health Organization (WHO)**
  - www.who.int
  - Provides global health information, including resources related to disabilities.
- **International Society for Autism Research**
  - www.autism-insar.org
  - Promotes and disseminates research related to autism worldwide.

5. Financial and Legal Resources

United States
- **National Disability Institute (NDI)**
  - www.nationaldisabilityinstitute.org
  - Provides resources and information about financial security for individuals with disabilities.
- **Disability Benefits Help**
  - www.disability-benefits-help.org
  - Offers guidance on obtaining Social Security Disability benefits.

International
- **Disability Rights International**
  - www.driadvocacy.org
  - Advocates for the rights of people with disabilities globally.
- **The World Bank: Disability Inclusion**
  - www.worldbank.org/en/topic/disability
  - Offers resources related to disability inclusion in economic development and policy.

6. Online Communities and Forums

United States
- **The Mighty**
  - www.themighty.com
  - An online community where parents and individuals can share their stories, experiences, and support.
- **Facebook Groups**
  - Many dedicated groups for parents of children with specific disabilities (e.g., Autism Support Groups, Down Syndrome Parents) can be found on Facebook, offering peer support and resources.

International
- **The Special Needs community on Reddit**
  - www.reddit.com/r/specialneeds
  - An online forum for discussing various aspects of raising children with special needs.

7. Publications

Books
- See Appendix A for a list of the books used within the SFN Mastermind Group weekly meetings, all written by SFN Mentor Fathers or others who were guests on the *SFN Dad To Dad Podcast*.
- For a more comprehensive list of books on fatherhood and disability, go to www.21stCenturyDads.org/additionalresources.

Journals and Articles
- *Exceptional Parent Magazine*: published monthly and available online for free: www.epmagazine.com
- *Journal of Special Education*: A peer-reviewed journal that publishes research on all aspects of special education. www.journals.sagepub.com/home/sed
- *Disability Studies Quarterly*: An interdisciplinary journal focusing on the study of disability. www.dsq-sds.org

8. Camps and Recreational Programs

United States

Here is a list of camps and recreational programs across the United States that cater to families raising children with disabilities and special needs. Each state is represented with at least two programs, along with the organization's website URLs for more information.

Alabama
1. Camp ASCCA (Alabama's Special Camp for Children and Adults): Offers year-round therapeutic recreation for children and adults with both physical and intellectual disabilities. https://www.campascca.org
2. The Exceptional Foundation: Located in Birmingham, The Exceptional Foundation provides year-round social and recreational activities for individuals with special needs, including a summer camp program. https://www.exceptionalfoundation.org

Alaska
1. Camp Fire Alaska: Offers inclusive camp programs that accommodate children with various disabilities, ensuring accessible activities and support. https://www.campfireak.org
2. Special Olympics Alaska: Provides year-round sports training and athletic competition for children and adults with intellectual disabilities, promoting physical fitness and community involvement. https://specialolympicsalaska.org

Arizona
1. Camp Not-A-Wheeze: A summer camp specifically designed for children with asthma, offering a traditional camp experience with medical supervision. https://www.campnotawheeze.org
2. Arizona Camp Sunrise and Sidekicks: Provides special programs for children who have or have had cancer and their siblings, including week-long camps and family retreats. https://www.azcampsunrise.org

Arkansas
1. Camp Aldersgate: Offers year-round programs for children with special needs, including summer medical camps and weekend respite programs. https://www.campaldersgate.net
2. Camp Quality Arkansas: Provides free camping experiences and year-round support for children with cancer and their families. https://www.campqualityusa.org/ar

California
1. Joni and Friends Family Retreats: A Global Christian Disability Ministry that provides week-long retreats throughout the U.S. and international locations. JAF also works with churches, synagogues and mosques to be more inclusive and accepting of people with disability and the Wheels for the World program which collects refurbishes and delivers wheelchairs around the world. https://joniandfriends.org

2. Camp Krem: Located in Boulder Creek, Camp Krem offers year-round programs for children and adults with developmental disabilities, including summer camps and travel programs. https://campingunlimited.org
3. The Painted Turtle: A medical specialty camp that provides a life-changing, free camp experience for children with serious medical conditions. https://www.thepaintedturtle.org

Colorado
1. Adam's Camp: Offers therapy, adventure, and family camps for children with developmental disabilities and their families. https://www.adamscamp.org
2. Roundup River Ranch: Provides free camp experiences for children with serious illnesses and their families in a medically-supported environment. https://roundupriverranch.org

Connecticut
1. Easterseals Camp Hemlocks: Offers accessible camping and recreational opportunities for children and adults with disabilities. https://www.easterseals.com/hartford/our-programs/camping-recreation
2. Camp Horizons: Provides summer camp programs, weekend events, and social programs for individuals with developmental disabilities. https://www.horizonsct.org

Delaware
1. Easterseals Camp Fairlee: Offers year-round camping and respite programs for children and adults with disabilities. https://www.campfairlee.com
2. Special Olympics Delaware: Provides year-round sports training and athletic competitions for individuals with intellectual disabilities. https://www.sode.org

Florida
1. Camp Boggy Creek: Offers year-round camp programs for children with serious illnesses and their families. https://www.boggycreek.org/
2. Easterseals Florida Camp Challenge: Provides camping experiences for children and adults with disabilities. https://florida.easterseals.com/get-support/areas-of-support/camp-and-recreation/camp-challenge

Georgia
1. Camp Twin Lakes: Partners with organizations to provide life-changing camp experiences for children with serious illnesses, disabilities, and other life challenges. https://camptwinlakes.org
2. Extra Special People (ESP) Camp: Offers summer camp programs for children and young adults with developmental disabilities. https://espyouandme.org/

Hawaii
1. Camp Imua: Provides a week-long recreational camp for children with special needs. https://discoverimua.com/camp/
2. Easterseals Hawaii: Offers various recreational programs for children with disabilities. https://www.eastersealshawaii.org/

Idaho

1. Camp Rainbow Gold: Offers camps for children diagnosed with cancer and their families. https://camprainbowgold.org/
2. Easterseals-Goodwill Northern Rocky Mountain: Provides recreational programs for children with disabilities. https://www.esgw.org/

Illinois

1. Timber Pointe Outdoor Center: Provides specialized outdoor recreational programs for individuals with disabilities and illnesses. https://www.timberpointeoutdoorcenter.com/
2. Jill's House: provides overnight camp for kids ages 6–17 with a diagnosed intellectual disability. https://jillshouse.org/programs/by-activities/weekend-adventures/
3. One in a Hundred Summer Camp: Helps children with challenges in establishing and maintaining friendships develop social language skills within a positive summer day camp experience. https://oneinahundredprogram.com/

Indiana

1. Camp Riley: Offers camp programs for youth with physical disabilities. https://bradfordwoods.iu.edu/Programs/rectherapy/campriley/index.html
2. Easterseals Crossroads: Provides recreational programs for children with disabilities. https://www.easterselascrossroads.org/
3. A Rosie Place for Children: Serves all ninety-two counties in the state of Indiana by providing respite care. https://arosieplace.org/

Iowa

1. Camp Courageous: A year-round respite care and recreational facility for individuals with disabilities. https://campcourageous.org/
2. Easterseals Iowa Camp Sunnyside: Offers camping and recreational programs for individuals with disabilities. https://ia.easterseals.com/get-support/areas-of-support/camp-sunnyside-services/summer-camp-sunnyside

Kansas

1. Camp Wood YMCA: Provides inclusive camp programs for children with disabilities. https://campwood.org/
2. Easterseals Capper Foundation: Offers recreational programs for children with disabilities. https://www.capper.org/

Kentucky

1. The Center for Courageous Kids: Offers free camp experiences for children with serious illnesses. https://www.courageouskids.org/
2. Easterseals West Kentucky: Provides recreational programs for children with disabilities. https://westkentucky.easterseals.com/

Louisiana

1. MedCamps of Louisiana: Provides free summer camp experiences for children with chronic illnesses and disabilities. https://medcamps.org/
2. Easterseals Louisiana: Offers recreational programs for children with disabilities. https://louisiana.easterseals.com/

Maine
1. Pine Tree Camp: Provides camp experiences for children and adults with disabilities. https://pinetreesociety.org/camp-home/
2. Camp CaPella: Offers recreational opportunities for children with disabilities. https://campcapella.org/

Maryland
1. Camp Greentop: Offers inclusive camp programs for children with and without disabilities. https://www.nps.gov/cato/planyourvisit/camp-greentop.htm
2. Easterseals DC MD VA: Provides recreational programs for children with disabilities. https://dcmdva.easterseals.com/

Massachusetts
1. Camp Arrowhead: Provides summer camp experiences for children with disabilities. https://camparrowhead.com/
2. Easterseals Massachusetts: Offers recreational programs for children with disabilities. https://massachusetts.easterseals.com/

Michigan
1. Camp Fish Tales: A barrier-free camp for children and adults with disabilities. https://campfishtales.org/
2. Easterseals Michigan: Provides recreational programs for children with disabilities. https://morc.easterseals.com/

Minnesota
1. True Friends Camps: Offers camp programs for children and adults with disabilities. https://truefriends.org/programs/camp/
2. Easterseals Minnesota: Provides recreational programs for children with disabilities. https://www.goodwilleasterseals.org/

Mississippi
1. Camp Lake Stephens: Offers inclusive camp programs for children with disabilities. https://www.camplakestephens.com/
2. Easterseals Mississippi: Provides recreational programs for children with disabilities. https://www.eastersealsms.org/

Missouri
1. Wonderland Camp: Provides a fun, educational camp experience for children, teenagers, and adults who have disabilities. https://wonderlandcamp.org/
2. Easterseals Midwest: Offers recreational programs for children with disabilities. https://midwest.easterseals.com/

Montana
1. Eagle Mount: Provides therapeutic recreational opportunities for people with disabilities. https://eaglemount.org/
2. Camp Māk-A-Dream: Offers cost-free camp experiences for children and young adults with cancer. https://www.campdream.org/

Nebraska
1. Camp CoHoLo: Provides a summer camp for children with cancer and blood disorders. https://camp-coholo.com/
2. Easterseals Nebraska: Offers recreational programs for children with disabilities. https://ne.easterseals.com/

Nevada
1. Camp Lotsafun: Offers summer camp for adults with disabilities, providing recreational and social opportunities. https://www.amplifylife.org/camp-lotsafun
2. Nevada PEP: Provides information on recreational programs and resources for families of children with disabilities. https://nvpep.org/

New Hampshire
1. Camp Allen: A summer camp offering programs for children and adults with developmental and physical challenges. https://www.campallennh.org/
2. Easterseals New Hampshire Camp Sno-Mo: Provides an overnight camp experience for children and young adults with disabilities. https://eastersealsnh.org/programs/camping-recreation/

New Jersey
1. Camp Merry Heart: Offers year-round camp programs for individuals with disabilities and special needs. https://www.merryheartchildrenscamp.org/
2. The Arc of New Jersey Family Institute: Provides resources and information on recreational programs for families of children with intellectual and developmental disabilities. https://www.thearcfamilyinstitute.org/

New Mexico
1. Camp Rising Sun: A summer camp for children with autism spectrum disorders, offering a traditional camp experience with necessary supports. https://www.groundworksnm.org/
2. New Mexico Autism Society: Provides information on recreational programs and resources for families of children with autism. https://nmautismsociety.org/

New York
1. Camp Anne: Offers a summer camp experience for children and adults with developmental disabilities. https://www.ahrcnyccamping.org/camp-anne
2. Camp Oakhurst: Provides summer camp sessions and year-round respite programs for children and adults with physical and developmental disabilities. https://www.campoakhurst.org/

North Carolina
1. Camp Royall: A camp for individuals with autism, offering year-round programs including summer camp, mini-camps, and family camps. https://www.autismsociety-nc.org/camp-royall/
2. Victory Junction: Provides camp experiences for children with serious illnesses and chronic medical conditions, including various disabilities. https://victoryjunction.org/

North Dakota
1. Elks Camp Grassick: A summer camp for children and adults with various disabilities, offering therapy and recreational activities. https://www.elkscampgrassick.com/
2. Anne Carlsen Center: Provides recreational programs and services for children with disabilities, including summer camps. https://annecarlsen.org/

Ohio
1. Camp Nuhop: Offers residential summer camp programs for children with learning disabilities, attention deficit disorders, and behavioral nuances. https://nuhop.org/
2. Recreation Unlimited: Provides year-round programs in sports, recreation, and education for individuals with disabilities and health concerns. https://recreationunlimited.org/

Oklahoma
1. Make Promises Happen: Offers camping experiences for individuals with disabilities, including summer camps and weekend retreats. https://www.camptwincedars.org/camps/make-promises-happen
2. The Center for Individuals with Physical Challenges: Provides adaptive recreational programs and activities for individuals with physical disabilities. https://www.tulsacenter.org/

Oregon
1. Mt. Hood Kiwanis Camp: Offers outdoor recreational programs for children and adults with disabilities, including summer camps. https://mhkc.org/
2. Camp Yakety Yak: A social skills day camp supporting children with special needs, including autism and communication disorders. https://www.campyaketyyak.org/

Pennsylvania
1. Easterseals Western and Central Pennsylvania Camps: Provides camp programs for children and adults with disabilities, offering various recreational activities. https://www.eastersealswcpa.org/
2. Camp Lee Mar: A private residential special needs camp for children and teenagers with mild to moderate learning and developmental challenges. https://www.leemar.com/

Rhode Island
1. Camp Surefire: A camp for children and teens with Type 1 diabetes, providing a traditional camp experience with medical support. https://campsurefire.org/
2. The Autism Project: Offers summer camp programs and other recreational activities for children with autism spectrum disorders. https://theautismproject.org/

South Carolina
1. Camp Burnt Gin: Offers summer sessions for children and young adults with physical disabilities and chronic illnesses. https://dph.sc.gov/health-wellness/child-teen-health/camp-burnt-gin/about-camp-burnt-gin

2. Camp Spearhead: Located in Marietta, Camp Spearhead provides residential summer camps and year-round programs for children and adults with special needs, focusing on social and recreational activities. https://campspearhead.org

South Dakota
1. Camp Gilbert: A week-long summer camp for children and teens with diabetes, offering education and support alongside traditional camp activities. https://www.campgilbert.com/
2. Joy Ranch: An accessible camp in Watertown that offers inclusive programs for individuals with various disabilities, including therapeutic horseback riding and adaptive sports. https://www.joyranchofsd.org/

Tennessee
1. Camp Conquest: A Christian camp in Cordova designed for children and adults with special needs and disabilities, offering activities like horseback riding, fishing, and zip-lining. https://www.campconquest.com/
2. Easterseals Tennessee Camp: Provides summer and weekend camping programs for children and adults with disabilities, focusing on recreation and social interaction. https://tn.easterseals.com/get-support/areas-of-support/recreational-camp

Texas
1. Camp CAMP (Children's Association for Maximum Potential): Offers year-round programs and summer camps for individuals with special needs, including a variety of recreational activities adapted to campers' abilities. https://campcamp.org/
2. Down Home Ranch: Provides camps and respite programs for individuals with intellectual and developmental disabilities, promoting social, educational, and vocational growth. https://www.downhomeranch.org/

Utah:
1. Camp Kostopulos (Camp K): Offers year-round and summer camps for children, teens, and adults with physical, developmental, and intellectual disabilities. Activities include a ropes course, horse riding, swimming, and fishing. https://www.campk.org/
2. National Ability Center: Provides over twenty adaptive recreation programs, including archery, rock climbing, high ropes courses, skiing, snowboarding, mountain biking, and watersports, tailored for individuals with disabilities. https://nationalabilitycenter.org/
3. Common Ground Outdoor Adventures: Provides adaptive equipment and support to enable people with disabilities to participate in outdoor recreation alongside their peers. Offers both in-person and virtual activities. https://www.cgadventures.org/
4. Autism Adventure Camp: A recreation-based summer program designed for 8 to 12-year-olds with level 1 autism spectrum disorder (ASD). Focuses on building self-care, social connections, and social skills. https://healthcare.utah.edu/hmhi/programs/autism-adventure-camp

Wisconsin:
1. Easterseals Wisconsin Camps, Camp Wawbeek: Offers programs for children, teens, young adults, and adults with disabilities. Activities include boating, fishing, hiking, and swimming. https://www.eastersealswisconsin.com/programs-services/camps/
2. Wisconsin Badger Camp: Hosts several camp sessions each summer for individuals with special needs, ranging from age 3 through adulthood. https://www.badgercamp.org/
3. Camp AweSum: Offers camps specifically designed for individuals and families affected by Autism Spectrum Disorders (ASD). https://ucci.org/camp-awesum-3/
4. Wisconsin Lions Camp: Provides camping experiences for children and adults who are blind or visually impaired, deaf or hard of hearing, or with intellectual disabilities including autism. https://www.wisconsinlionscamp.com/

Wyoming:
1. Camp Carpe Diem: Designed for youth to experience a variety of new tasks, develop leadership skills, and build self-confidence. https://campcarpediem.com/
2. The Arc of Natrona County Summer Camp: Offers a week-long day camp on Casper Mountain each July, providing outdoor activities, games, crafts, and a petting zoo. https://arcofnatronacounty.org/
3. Teton Valley Ranch Camp: Provides a residential summer camp experience for kids ages 11–16, offering activities like horseback riding, backpacking, and outdoor adventures in the Wyoming wilderness. https://www.tvrcamp.org/

District of Columbia:
1. Discovery Inclusion Camp: A summer camp experience for children with disabilities ages 6–10, integrated into the DC Parks and Recreation Discovery Camp programs. https://dpr.dc.gov/page/therapeutic-recreation-camps
2. Kids in Action: An adaptive sports and social activities program for children and young adults with disabilities and their siblings. Offers a range of adapted sports, social, and health-based activities focusing on each child's goals and strengths. https://www.childrensnational.org/get-care/departments/rehabilitation-specialized-care/community-and-rec-therapy/kids-in-action
3. Camp Accomplish: An inclusive summer camp open to youth aged 5–18, serving campers with and without disabilities and chronic health conditions. https://campaccomplish.org/
4. Jill's House: provides rest renewal, and relationships for kids with intellectual disabilities and their families. https://jillshouse.org/

International

Finding specialized camps and recreational programs for families raising children with disabilities and special needs can be challenging, especially across multiple countries. While comprehensive information for each country may not be readily available, here are some resources and programs that cater to such families in countries Special Fathers Network has a presence:

Canada:
1. Tamwood International Camps: Offers engaging language and activity camps at various locations in Canada, providing a summer of fun and learning. https://tamwood.com/camps/
2. Easter Seals Canada: Provides accessible summer camp programs tailored for children with disabilities, focusing on inclusivity and personal development. https://easterseals.ca/en/
3. Camp Awakening: Offers outdoor recreational programs for youth with physical disabilities, promoting independence and personal growth. https://www.kidsprograms.ca/location/camp-awakening/

Cayman Islands:
1. Inclusive Community Life by Inclusion Cayman: Supports families in accessing recreational activities and community events of their choice. They also assist community and recreation providers in successfully including individuals with disabilities. https://inclusioncayman.ky/inclusive-community-life
2. Caribbean Marine Ecology Camp by Central Caribbean Marine Institute (CCMI): offers a week-long summer camp for high school students aged 13–17. The program includes scuba diving, snorkeling, and learning about tropical marine ecology and conservation. While not exclusively for children with disabilities, CCMI emphasizes inclusivity and may accommodate special needs upon request. https://reefresearch.org/our-work/education/summer-camps/

Cuba:
1. CubaHeal's Child Development and Rehabilitation Programs: CubaHeal offers personalized medical programs for the evaluation and treatment of various developmental disabilities, including autism spectrum disorder, cerebral palsy, and intellectual disabilities. https://cubaheal.com/
2. Asociación Nacional de Sordos de Cuba (ANSOC): The Cuban National Association of the Deaf provides support and resources for individuals with hearing impairments. They offer various programs aimed at social inclusion and empowerment of the deaf community in Cuba. https://www.mtss.gob.cu/asociaciones/ansoc
3. Special Education System in Cuba: The Cuban government has implemented a comprehensive special education system to ensure that all children with disabilities receive appropriate education. https://cubaplusmagazine.com/en/health-medicine/special-education-cuba-equal-opportunity-all.html

England:
1. Calvert Trust: Specializes in outdoor adventure activities for people with disabilities, offering family breaks that include various inclusive activities. https://calvertlakes.org.uk/
2. Over The Wall: Provides free activity camps for children with health challenges and their families, aiming to build confidence and support. https://www.otw.org.uk/
3. The Wingate Centre: Offers residential camps and recreational activities designed for children and young adults with disabilities. https://www.thewingatecentre.co.uk/booking

France:
1. APF Evasion: Organizes holiday camps for children and adults with physical disabilities, providing various recreational activities in accessible settings. https://apf-evasion.org/
2. ANAE: Offers adapted holiday camps for individuals with disabilities, focusing on inclusive recreational experiences. https://www.anae.asso.fr/
3. UFCV: Provides specialized holiday camps for children with disabilities, ensuring accessible facilities and tailored programs. https://vacances-adaptees.ufcv.fr/le-catalogue-printemps-ete-2025-est-arrive-decouvrez-nos-sejours/

Germany:
1. Special Olympics Germany: Provides year-round sports training and athletic competition for children and adults with intellectual disabilities, offering opportunities to develop physical fitness and experience joy. https://www.specialolympics.org/programs/europe-eurasia/germany
2. Bundesverband für körper- und mehrfachbehinderte Menschen e.V. (bvkm): Offers recreational programs and camps for children with multiple disabilities, focusing on inclusive activities. https://bvkm.de/
3. Aktion Mensch: Supports various inclusive recreational projects and camps for families with children with disabilities across Germany. https://www.aktion-mensch.de/

Iceland:
1. Reykjavík Summer Activities for Children and Adolescents: The City of Reykjavík offers a variety of summer programs, including after-school activities, youth centers, sailing courses, summer camps, sports courses, and riding courses. These programs are designed to be inclusive and cater to children with diverse needs. reykjavik.is https://reykjavik.is/en/news/2024/courses-and-summer-activities-children-and-adolescents?utm
2. Þroskafjör—Empowering the Development of Refugee Children: en.hafnarfjordur.is
3. Summer Camps for Disabled Children: In various locations across Iceland, summer camps are available for disabled children. These camps are run by local authorities, nonprofit organizations, or individuals, offering tailored activities to meet the needs of children with disabilities. https://island.is/en/rights-of-people-with-disabilities-to-general-services-and-assistance?utm
4. Icelandic Disability Alliance: is an umbrella organization of forty-three associations of people with disabilities in Iceland. https://www.obi.is/about-obi/

India:
1. Tamana: Provides summer camps and recreational programs for children with autism and other developmental disabilities, focusing on skill development and social interaction. https://tamana.ngo/
2. AADI (Action for Ability Development and Inclusion): Offers recreational activities and camps for children with disabilities, promoting inclusion and personal growth. https://aadi-india.org/
3. SPJ Sadhana School: Conducts summer camps focusing on arts, crafts, and other recreational activities tailored for children with special needs. https://spjsadhanaschool.org/

Israel:
1. Shalva: Offers inclusive summer camps and recreational programs for children with disabilities, providing various activities and support services. https://www.shalva.org/main/national-center/
2. ADI Negev: founded by Doron Almog and named after his son Eran, ADI Negev is a rehabilitation village and community where people from diverse backgrounds and all levels of ability can live, heal and grow together. https://adi-il.org/adi-negev/
3. AKIM Israel: Provides recreational programs and camps for children with intellectual disabilities, focusing on social integration and personal development. https://akimisrael.com/
4. Beit Issie Shapiro: Offers various recreational and therapeutic programs for children with disabilities, including summer camps and after-school activities. https://beitissie.org.il/en/

Japan:
1. Solaputi Kids' Camp: Part of the SeriousFun Children's Network, it offers recreational experiences tailored for children with serious illnesses. The camp provides a supportive environment where children can engage in various activities designed to accommodate their medical needs. https://www.solaputi.jp/en/
2. Nippon Agoonoree: Organized by the Scout Association of Japan, it is a Scouting jamboree specifically designed for young people with disabilities. Held every four years, this event offers participants the opportunity to engage in various Scouting activities in an inclusive environment. https://www.scout.or.jp/member/agoonoree
3. EdVenture Niseko: Located in Hokkaido, it provides unique outdoor programs that connect children from around the world. While not exclusively for children with disabilities, their inclusive approach and diverse activities may be suitable for some families. It's recommended to contact them directly to discuss specific needs. https://www.edventureniseko.com/
4. Ashinaga Rainbow House: an organization that supports orphaned children, including those who have lost parents due to illness or disaster. The Rainbow House offers programs and camps that provide emotional support and recreational activities for children facing such challenges. https://www.ashinaga.org/

5. Japan Barrier-Free Association: Organizes recreational programs and camps for children with disabilities, promoting accessibility and inclusion. https://barrierfreejapan.com/2025/01/25/farm-welfare-links-for-disabled-employment-expand-in-japan/
6. National Rehabilitation Center for Children with Disabilities: Provides various recreational and therapeutic programs, including camps, for children with disabilities. https://www.rehab.go.jp/english/index.html

Kenya:
1. Wendo Retreat and Resource Centre's Special Needs Camp: This camp offers children aged 5 and above with developmental disabilities the opportunity to experience various beneficial activities. http://wendoretreat.org/
2. Jesuit Refugee Service (JRS) Special Needs Program in Kakuma: JRS promotes inclusive education for persons living with disabilities in Kakuma refugee camp. They provide functional skills training, rehabilitation, and capacity building for caregivers. https://www.jrsusa.org/
3. The Action Foundation's Medical Camps: The Action Foundation organizes free pediatric medical camps offering consultations, diagnosis, and treatment for children with disabilities. These camps aim to support the holistic health, growth, and development of children in low-resource communities. http://theactionfoundationkenya.org/
4. Kupenda for the Children: Kupenda (meaning "love" in Kiswahili) is a nonprofit organization that develops disability advocacy and training programs to transform negative beliefs surrounding disability. They focus on educating families and communities about the rights of children with disabilities and how to support them. https://kupenda.org/

Norway:
1. Ridderrennet: Hosts an annual winter sports week for individuals with disabilities, including families, offering skiing and other activities. https://www.ridderrennet.com/
2. Hurdal Syn- og Mestringssenter: Offers recreational programs and camps for visually impaired children and their families, focusing on outdoor activities. https://www.blindeforbundet.no/tilbud-kurs-og-arrangementer/syn-og-mestringssentrene

Poland:
1. Little Explorers Summer Camps: Provides engaging and exciting activities for children with disabilities, focusing on artistic workshops and personal development. https://www.globalgiving.org/projects/little-explorers/
2. Fundacja Aktywnej Rehabilitacji (FAR): Organizes camps and recreational programs for children with physical disabilities, promoting active rehabilitation. https://far.org.pl/
3. Stowarzyszenie Na Tak: Offers various recreational activities and camps for children with intellectual disabilities, focusing on social integration. https://natak.pl/

Tanzania:

1. Faraja School: is the only residential primary school in Kilimanjaro, Tanzania, where children with special needs receive an excellent K-7 education. https://www.farajaschool.org/
2. BCC Special Needs Centres (Building a Caring Community): a network of special needs centers supported by the Evangelical Lutheran Church and partners that provides education, therapy, life skills training, and community involvement for children and young adults with disabilities (ages ~3–22). https://tanzaniavolunteers.com/bcc-centers/
3. Special Needs Children Camp (Nyota Foundation): a special needs children camp hosted by the Nyota Foundation, specifically designed as a camp experience for children with various disabilities. https://nyotafoundation.co.tz/special-needs-children-camp/

Uganda:

1. Angel's Center for Children with Special Needs: supports children with intellectual disabilities and their families through rehabilitation programs including early learning, therapy, livelihoods and advocacy in Uganda. https://angelscentre.org/
2. Kyaninga Child Development Centre (KCDC): provides specialized assessment, treatment, education, and support to children with disabilities. They offer therapy, rehabilitation, and training programs, along with community-based rehabilitation and inclusive education initiatives. https://www.kyaningacdc.org/
3. The Recreation Project: Based in Gulu, The Recreation Project uses adventure-based counseling to equip young people and their families with life skills. They offer programs like the Climbing Club and primary school initiatives, focusing on resilience and personal development through outdoor activities. https://www.therecreationproject.org/
4. Ashinaga Uganda: Ashinaga Uganda provides emotional and educational support to orphans, including those with disabilities. They run programs such as the Rainbow House, which offers psychological support and recreational activities, and the Kokoro Juku, a residential facility supporting students' educational pursuits. https://www.ashinaga.org/en/ashinaga-global-network/ashinaga-uganda/
5. Sanyuka Camp (SeriousFun Children's Network): Part of the SeriousFun Children's Network, Sanyuka Camp offers recreational experiences tailored for children with serious illnesses and disabilities. https://www.seriousfun.org/
6. Joy for Children Uganda: This organization implements projects supporting children with disabilities, including inclusive education initiatives. https://www.hasanah.org/nonprofits/joy-for-children-uganda

Other Global Programs:

1. Special Olympics: Provides year-round sports training and athletic competitions for children and adults with intellectual disabilities across more than one hundred countries. https://www.specialolympics.org/
2. Global Volunteers: Offers family volunteering opportunities worldwide, including programs that support children with disabilities. https://globalvolunteers.org/

3. European Network for Independent Living (ENIL): Supports independent living for individuals with disabilities across Europe, including recreational programs. https://enil.eu/

9. Technology and Apps

Assistive Technology
- AT3 Center: Provides information on assistive technology products and resources. https://exploreat.net/
- Apps for Children with Special Needs: Many apps are available to aid learning and communication, including Proloquo2Go, ABCmouse, and TouchChat.

Online Tools
- Khan Academy: Offers free educational resources for children of all abilities. https://www.khanacademy.org/

10. Local Resources

Community Resources
- Local School Districts: Many school districts offer resources, support services, and IEP guidance for children with special needs.
- Community Centers: Local community centers may have programs and services tailored for families with special needs.
- Local Libraries: Many libraries offer resources, workshops, and story times specifically designed for children with disabilities.

Finding Local Resources
- 211: A resource hotline that can connect families to local services and support groups based on their needs.
- Local Health Departments: They can provide information on early intervention programs, developmental screenings, and local services.

Conclusion

This primer of resource appendix aims to empower parents raising children with special needs and disabilities. By accessing these organizations, support groups, educational tools, and community resources, families can navigate their journeys with greater confidence, support, and knowledge. The path of parenting a child with special needs may present unique challenges, but it also offers profound opportunities for growth, understanding, and connection. With the right resources, parents can build a strong foundation for their children, fostering resilience, independence, and a lasting legacy of love and support.

About David Hirsch

David Hirsch is the father of five, a seasoned financial advisor, and one of the country's leading, most outspoken advocates for children and fathers. He's the founder of two fatherhood nonprofits, author, TEDx Speaker, and host of the *Special Fathers Network Dad To Dad Podcast*, now with more than 400 episodes.

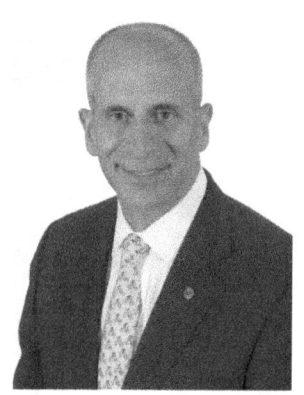

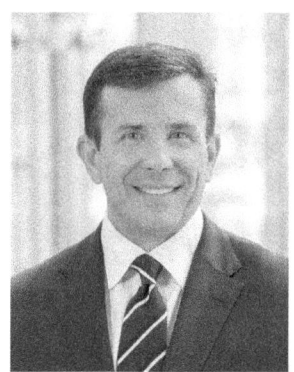

About John F. Crowley

John F. Crowley is a father, president, and CEO of Biotechnology Innovation Organization (BIO) as well as former longtime CEO of Amicus Therapeutics. John is also an author and speaker. Perhaps most importantly, he found a cure for Pompe Disease that saved the lives of two of his children and untold others.

www.ingramcontent.com/pod-product-compliance
Lightning Source LLC
LaVergne TN
LVHW011928070526
838202LV00054B/4544